Training
Tips and Routines

The Best of Joe Weider's

MUSCLE
& FITNESS
Training
Tips and Routines

Contemporary Books, Inc.
Chicago

Library of Congress Cataloging in Publication Data

Main entry under title:

The best of Joe Weider's *Muscle & Fitness:*
training tips and routines.

    1. Weight lifting—Addresses, essays, lectures.
2. Bodybuilding—Addresses, essays, lectures.
I. Weider, Joe.
GV546.B47   1981   646.7′5   80-70630
ISBN 0-8092-5911-7   AACR2
ISBN 0-8092-5910-9 (pbk.)

All photos courtesy of the IFBB

Published by Contemporary Books, Inc.
180 North Michigan Avenue, Chicago, Illinois 60601
Manufactured in the United States of America
Library of Congress Catalog Card Number: 80-70630
International Standard Book Number: 0-8092-5911-7 (cloth)
                                   0-8092-5910-9 (paper)

Published simultaneously in Canada by
Beaverbooks, Ltd.
150 Lesmill Road
Don Mills, Ontario M3B 2T5
Canada

Contents

1 TRAINING TIPS

3 The Weider System: Development of a
Training Philosophy
by Joe Weider

8 Mind Power in Bodybuilding
by Pete Grymkowski

11 Bodybuilding Workouts: How Often Is Best
by Larry Scott

16 The Thinking Man's Repetition
by Casey Viator

21 Updating High-Intensity Methods
by Mike Mentzer

29 Secrets of Getting Ripped
by Tom Platz

32 The Reverse Gravity Principle of Training
by Joe Weider

35 Iso-Tension Concentration for Olympia
Muscularity
by Joe Weider

38 Running and the Bodybuilder
by Bill Dobbins

41 My Way
by Ed Corney

45 Cold Cure for Muscle Injury
by Dr. Franco Columbu

48 Machines: Scientific Shortcut to Success?
by Bill Dobbins

52 Machines: A Pitfall on the Way to Progress?
by George Elder

55 ROUTINES

57 Beginner's Bodybuilding Training
by Andreas Cahling

62 Second-Stage Training Boost
by Andreas Cahling

65 Advanced Training
by Andreas Cahling

68 Lou Ferrigno: Working to Break the 60-Inch
Chest Barrier
by Lou Ferrigno as told to Bill Reynolds

73 My Definitive Biceps Workout
*by Arnold Schwarzenegger as told to Bill
Reynolds*

79 The Key to Big Arms
by Boyer Coe

82 Back: How to Build It
by Robby Robinson

86 Franco: Updating Deltoid Training
by Dr. Franco Columbu

90 Building Muscular Thighs
by Samir Bannout

93 Calves—You Can!
by Chris Dickerson

97 Indirect Muscle Stimulation . . . Not
Training the Forearms: Sometimes It's
Better
by Mike Mentzer

99 The Ripped Waistline
by Danny Padilla

103 Power Exercises for Bodybuilders
by Joe Weider

TRAINING TIPS

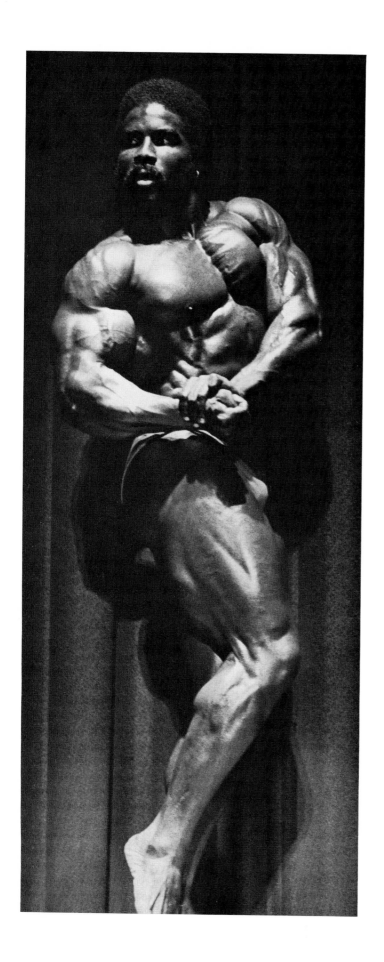

"The Weider Principles were developed to take the bodybuilder progressively step by step into advanced training. They were breakouts from static methods and breakthroughs to unceasing muscular growth."

—Robby Robinson

The Weider System
Development of a Training Philosophy

by Joe Weider

From the late 1880s to the late 1930s, weight training was a stiff, measured discipline. It took its cue from the organized Germans and the conservative British, entered America through conformist Alan Calvert and eventually landed with the reactionary York organization.

The distillate workout at that time consisted of three training sessions weekly, no more no less, each workout comprising nine to 12 basic exercises and only one set of eight to 10 reps at the start for each exercise. Instructions were to increase one rep weekly until 12 to 15 were accomplished at which time three to five pounds were added and the process repeated again with eight to 10 reps. This litany occurred every Monday, Wednesday and Friday. To deviate a day might have negated its blessing.

It had its good points: basic exercises worked all the muscles of the body, the progressive resistance principle was observed and time for recuperation was allowed. It also helped organize a person's training habits. Well and good, but what it didn't do was take into consideration those intrinsic qualities of individual strength, recuperative power, body type and genetic endowment. It froze him in a beginner's program. He remained a perpetual sophomore with no further curriculum. He became a victim of the adaptation response and the law of diminishing returns. His efforts eventually became boring as progress appeared hopeless. He strayed, baffled by the realization that simple labor alone did not suffice, or was not rewarded.

There were mustangs—guys like Grimek, Horvath and some others—strength oriented musclemen who went into weightlifting or powerlifting. The heavy weights generated a further muscle building response that had eluded most of the fraternity of bodybuilders. It happened to be a step in the right direction, but no one seemed able to corral that runaway power and tame it in a way to build muscular detail.

Having been a weightlifter myself, I pondered the problem. I had set some provincial lifting records and had also become a strong amateur wrestler. While still in my teens, I began to question the efficacy of the existing training methods. It was not unusual at that time to see a genetically endowed man do in two months of training what it took another man of lesser potential two years to do. With today's state of the art that would never happen. Now in two years, the average guy can almost become a superman.

I was a rebel when I was young, but I was imbued with a deep sense of responsibility. When I was 11 years old, I had to leave school to help keep my family together financially during the Great Depression of the 1930s. Out of necessity I became intuitive and imaginative, so when I eventually landed in weight training, I instinctively peeked around corners. I was incapable of accepting anything at face value.

I began to examine the old training methods and realized that they didn't work. The system said work out Monday, Wednesday and Friday. There were times that maybe I didn't feel like working out on a Monday, too beat, but by Tuesday I was raring to go again. Since it was sacrilegious to work out on Tuesday, I helplessly let the day pass by.

Also, you were allowed to increase your poundages no more than five pounds every month or so. If your progress was such that you could have added 10 pounds more, you were again stymied. Before long I'd had a stomach full of that. I then wrote an article called "Routines Are Made To Be Broken" in which I railed against the tyranny of tradition. Routines were made to serve, I said, not to be served.

During the 1940s when the whole world went through upheaval and change, I had begun to develop a certain spirit of reconstruction. I had the opportunity to train and be with many of the emerging bodybuilding stars of that era. I studied their methods and found that they were doing things in their workouts *instinctively* which they were unaware of, little cheats and turns that expedited the movement of weights. I remember an incident with Clarence Ross, a superstar of

"Some equipment companies, and even some ill-advised bodybuilders think they can master the nature of muscle growth with metal devices, drugs and techniques that outrage the laws of muscular growth. Like the alchemists and magicians of the middle ages, they too must fail."

"Sensitivity and intuition along with logic and experiment were tied together to produce the instinctive way of training."

"Only the bodybuilding artist can build mass, definition and shape all at once."
—Rick Wayne

that period. I watched him do a set of barbell curls, 10 reps with 165 pounds, but I noticed he had to cheat them. That was a heavy weight of course. At the same time one of Ross' students who was copying the star, only with a lighter weight, got a scolding from his mentor for cheating his curls.

Ross told him to do them strict, no cheating. I was thinking how entirely old-world that advice was. As Clancy returned to the bar for another set, I suggested he do the curls the same way he told the student, strict. With an awkward effort he could do only four strict reps, not the 10 reps he did before. Only then did I make Clancy aware that he was using cheating and forced reps methods in some of his movements, one of the big reasons for his well-known bodybuilding strength.

The same thing happened in weightlifting. Many champions had discovered that by cleaning the weight to the shoulder with the entire body arched forward they could heave-press a weight rapidly overhead by jerking the body erect without even bending the knees. That trick, in fact, caused the elimination of the

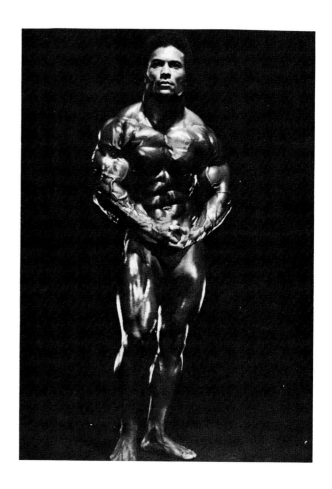

Two Arm Press from Olympic lifting competion. But for a period of several years it was enough to fool and confuse the judges. The lifters also instinctively used a slight pushout as they snatched, a movement contrary to the perfectly vertical pull required by the lifting rules.

Cheating and forcing were used by lifters, yet everyone was advised to use strict styles according to tradition. Unaware that they were so disorganized, they truly believed in the rules. Stated another way: There's nothing that says you can't beat your wife and believe in God also. In short, instinct never suffers the confusion of reason. Those weightlifters instinctively learned the best way to lift the most weight, legislated rules notwithstanding.

For a period of time, weight training and weightlifting were in a mess: No regimented method was devised that worked. Weightlifting articles used to be written stressing technique, how to get the weight up. Almost nothing was written on power assistance exercises, improving the total muscular structure and building strength outside the required channels.

Neither did that fault lie entirely with the lifters and bodybuilders. Athletic coaches in general were blind and obstinate about weight training, thinking it would make their athletes musclebound. It wasn't until the Russian athletes who were trained with power assistance exercises began beating the pants off us that we finally woke up to the value of weight training in all sports.

Weight-trained East European boxers are still knocking the heads off our boxers whose coaches to this day do not recognize the benefits of assistance power exercises to build greater hitting power. Today Muhammed Ali works on a strength-building program which should convince American boxing coaches to follow suit. Old systems take a long time to die.

When I began publishing over 35 years ago, I was adrift on a sea fraught with peril. I had set my course to follow the most direct route to that distant land of scientific training fact in hopes of returning with the spice of evidence that would make weight training palatable. In landfalls along the way, the natives were not always friendly. Those bodybuilding champs eyed me with suspicion when I asked to examine their training methods and didn't fall over when I suggested they test-try some new training idea. I fell under attack by some people in the business. After all, rebels are seldom invited to dinner by the entrenched owners.

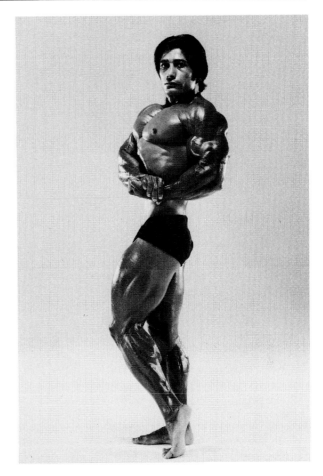

"Through instinctive training, the bodybuilder becomes the true artist, the requisite for stardom."
—Danny Padilla

Eventually I succeeded. The real meaning of my journey could not be misinterpreted. The evidence showed in every issue of *Muscle & Fitness.* I pampered the game, and my fondness for it won me wide support. People offered to help me develop the Weider System. Some of these good bodybuilders were banned by the AAU for doing this, their careers ruined by bigots. Some lost deserved titles while others were not permitted to enter AAU events. They were guilty of associating with me and of trying to increase the knowledge of the sport. Nevertheless I finally was able to convince enough champions and near champions to cooperate with me to test my techniques.

I followed a three-step method in developing all the techniques:

1. By training with weights myself in all forms, I was able to develop an intuition that sensed exactly what worked for me. I also had the opportunity to train with the champs along with

hundreds of other hard-training bodybuilders. I could see and feel the results. I saw the relationship between effort and recuperation. I felt that effort and recuperation were two distinct parts of training, yet conjoined physiologically.

2. The character of the effort and the recuperative force at work needed a collective name. Forced Reps and Supersets were both different methods, for example, varying in degree of intensity of effort and length of rest between sets and even between repetitions.

3. By giving each concept a name, I knew it would be easier to remember. Each name had to be a thumbnail sketch of the system. When you said "Forced Reps" you understood it meant going beyond the threshold of regular effort, beyond simple fatigue into the area of exhaustion. By naming them it was easier to unify them. That is what I called the "knot" that tied all the principles together, that enabled the Weider Instinctive Principle to be developed: In this way, a core sense and somatic intuition along with logic and experiment were tied together to produce the instinctive way of training.

I once had a long list of the different principles that were developed. Some got absorbed along the way, combined with other concepts, and the final outcome is the list of major principles as we know them today: Supersets, Tri Sets, Giant Sets, Peak-Contraction, Forced Reps, Overload Method, Reverse Gravity System, Split System, Double-Split System, Cheating and Quality Training.

All of these principles were created for one reason—to gradually increase workout intensity in order to build greater power and larger muscular mass faster. With the early methods, progress slowed considerably after the first 30 days. One of the first techniques we came up with to break free from that ancient tether was Supersets. It practically eliminated the rest period between sets, a mighty innovation, electronic compared to the spring-loaded timing procedures of old. Supersets pushed training along with new fuel for growth.

But even Supersets reached a point of diminishing returns, and in the search for another breakthrough we developed Tri Sets and then Giant Sets. Thus the process continued, each new method taking us another step further on the road to intensity of training, a kind of carrot we had to keep chasing.

Some of the methods I developed applied to

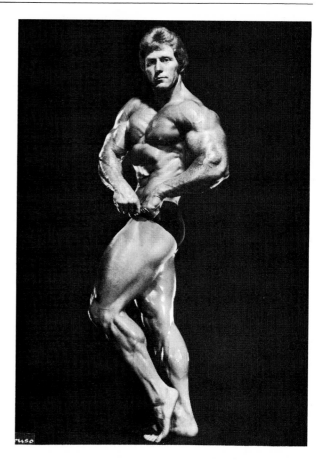

"Mastery of the various techniques along with learning the art of recuperation provide the spring board to instinctive training and ultimate progress."

"The bodybuilder, like the law student or medical student, must master his subject before he can utilize the knowledge to be creative."

—Ken Waller

overall workouts while others were developed to increase the intensity of working individual muscle groups. For instance, from regular biceps curls, we advanced to the Superset, then on to Cheating, Peak Contraction and Forced Reps— each subsequent method designed either to intensify or isolate effort to build mass and shape respectively.

Each method was built on the previous one. When one served its purpose and exhausted itself, we compounded it with a new one. The old one was not discarded. You don't give a beginner Supersets. Nor do you give an intermediate bodybuilder the Double-Split System. The Systems for the most part are used in a logical order, each geared to expedite muscle growth, to maintain momentum, like stages of a rocket.

Each method served a different purpose. Some were created to develop parts of a muscle through isolation, others for building muscle mass, or still others for taking advantage of the physiological recuperative power of muscle as it grows. Others may offer combined effects like both definition and mass.

Each Weider Principle has a life of its own in the game. Each continues to grow, nourished by new input from champions using it, or through the ever-increasing outpourings of scientific research.

Intensity is the condition that prevails over all these principles to form the knot that binds them together for the common purpose—steady muscular growth. That is the keynote of the Weider System, eliminating stagnation and hastening progress.

The methods are geared like a transmission that permits the beginner to start in low gear and shift up as he gains momentum. With a knowledge of the methods and the names given to them, he can pick what he thinks will work for him. Eventually, after several years, he should be able to function in the realm of Instinctive Training. That means he will still work with the different Weider methods that he learned as an intermediate bodybuilder but with greater sophistication. He will learn to intensify and pace. He will have a greater backlog with which to make comparisons. He will simply be a more fully loaded computer. But it will be his holistic intelligence that sets the programs for the instinct, so to speak.

I have found that the superstars like Zane, Mentzer, Ferrigno or Padilla listen most carefully or search most avidly for any idea that may help them gain the slightest bit. They are humbled by years of training and by both the joys of winning and disappointment of losing physique titles which give their lives force.

I have tried to explain how and why the Weider System was developed. I explained how they were tested and how they grew. I explained the meaning of the *knot* that pulled all these methods together to form the Instinctive Principle, catalyzed by intensity of effort.

Now well into the fourth generation, bodybuilders have been using these techniques. Training has become highly refined and more penetrating now due to the latest advances in sports medicine. Bodies are getting better, faster. Third place winners today would never have lost a contest 15 years ago. Times they are a-changing.

So am I in my attitudes toward training. I intend to keep all avenues open for the advancement of the sport. We all have *Muscle & Fitness* magazine to work with. You can depend on anything worthwhile to appear on these pages.

Lastly, I want all my student friends to realize the fact that working out in the gym is only half of your training—recuperation is the other half. You have to build recuperative power. It isn't something that comes overnight with eight hours sleep. It is truly more involved.

You must come to the realization that when you are not in the gym working out, when your body is recuperating, your workout is still going on. Successful training consists of two elements: the ultimate workout and total recuperation.

Mind Power in Bodybuilding

by Pete Grymkowski

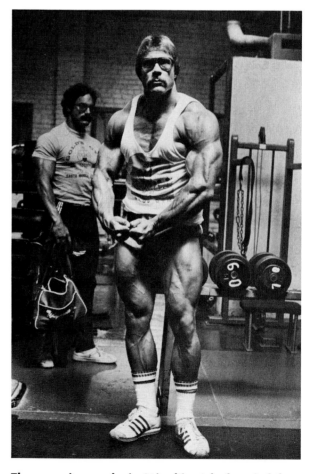

The excercises are basic. It is ultimately the mind that makes a champion.

Robby Robinson stands in front of a mirror at Gold's Gym. He tenses the incredible leg biceps, twists the corrugated torso, flexes the iron biceps. And as he does this, he looks—not only with his eyes, but with the mind's eye. He sees not only how he is, but what he will someday be. He is molding an image in his thoughts that he will force his body to copy. He is creating himself with mind power.

Nothing you can do with your mind will create a great physique unless you are willing to put in hours of strenuous effort in the gym. But, if the proper mental machinery is not put into action, your development will reach a sticking point and go no further.

"Determination isn't enough to make a champion," says Mr. Universe Tom Platz. "To me, it seems more like desperation. You can't just 'want to'—you have to 'have to!'" Tom works hard in the gym, but like Robby, he knows it takes more than physical effort to produce superhuman results. So he, too, cultivates a clear image in his mind depicting how he would like—no, how he is determined—to look.

"Your mind controls everything," Tom is

certain. "It even controls how you cut up. I've tried it. With enough mental effort, you can make yourself into anything that your genetic endowment permits."

But it is one thing to believe in the power of the mind, and quite another to actually harness that power. Just as in the performance of exercises, technique plays an important role in making use of the mind. And confirmation is coming to bodybuilding from other sports that these techniques are real, of practical benefit and can be learned.

"Visualization" is one new and important technique for bringing the power of the mind to bear on sports performance. This involves mentally rehearsing each movement and effort involved in the execution of sports technique. Tests have shown that the body is involved in even that which seems to be purely mental effort. If you visualize yourself running or throwing a ball or the like, your muscles will involuntarily tense as if you were actually performing those movements. It is believed that visualization actually helps develop the neural habits that are required for the precise control of sports activities. By constant repetition in the mind, you make those movements automatic.

Visualization can also be auditory as well as visual and muscular. But however it is done, it requires the utmost concentration, a necessary habit in itself. But concentration can be both a help and a hindrance. If you concentrate so hard that you become tense and anxious, your performance will suffer accordingly. Therefore, teachers of visualization stress that these exercises should also be accompanied by relaxation.

Relaxation increases the benefits you acquire from the mental exercises, and teaches you to associate the activity you are visualizing with a calm and relaxed frame of mind. Therefore, when it comes time to put what you have visualized into practice, you are more likely to remain relaxed and confident.

The most familiar application of visualization to bodybuilding is in the formation of goals. Top bodybuilders have a clear image of what kind of physique they are working toward. Whether it is Robby, Tom Platz, Frank Zane or any other champion, what they have achieved is, for them, only a reflection of the ideal proportions and development that stands out clear in their imaginations.

"When I pose in front of the mirror," Robby explains, "I am seeing both what is there and what I want to be there. The mind and body are connected. Just as you force your body to develop by subjecting it to the stress of training, you have to train your mind as well. You have to condition it to accept the inevitability of ultimate achievement. To get past a certain point, your mental image of yourself has to grow before your body will."

Frank Zane agrees that the mind has great influence on the body. "There's no doubt about it," he declares "if you have a clear enough idea as to how you want your body to grow—and you put in your time at the gym—it will be influenced by your mental imagery. I don't know exactly how this works, but I am convinced it does."

Merely having an image clear in your mind is not enough. It has to be a true image, one that relates to your actual physical gifts, natural proportions, and admits to your weak points as well as your strengths. It may be an idealization, but it must be based on accurate observation. Danny Padilla is never going to be tall, no matter what else he achieves. Nor could Frank Zane develop the thickness of a Mike Mentzer. Every bodybuilder is a prisoner of his genetic endowment. To ignore that is to stray from visualization into the world of fantasy.

Also, the idealized image and the facts reflected in the mirror must be fairly compared. That is hard for some bodybuilders. Why else would otherwise top-rated competitors continue year after year with outstanding and well-known weaknesses without altering their training routines accordingly? Habit has something to do with it. It is hard, after years of effort resulting in some success, to admit to failure in certain areas and force yourself to practically start over. A real weakness takes years to convert into a strength. A Mr. Universe or Mr. Olympia competitor has already put in the years and finds it difficult to accept such a setback.

Mental attitude becomes important from the time a novice bodybuilder first sets foot in a gym. First, there is desire, strong enough to make him go through the endless hours of repetitions and the agony of pushing himself beyond endurance. Then there is discipline of keeping up these efforts month after month, year after year, and the harshness of sticking to diets that rarely satisfy the appetite. And, in the gym, the thing that differentiates the top contender from the also-ran is concentration and the ability to get the most out of training efforts.

"I concentrate on each individual muscle,"

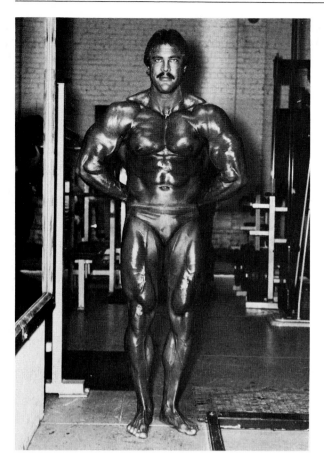

"Use these mind blowing techniques along with your overload workouts, and I'm sure your muscle gains will soar to new heights."

—Pete Grymkowski

Robby says, "I want to isolate and punish each one, each fiber if I can." Tom Platz, on the other hand, does not concentrate on the individual muscles so much as he tries to generate an intensity so great that he will blast his muscles into growing with the effort. "I can tell after the workout how well I have done," he says. "I feel spent, exhausted and used up. But it's a good feeling, one of accomplishment. When I feel that way I know I have gone beyond the barriers and my body will have to respond."

"Actually," Frank Zane believes, "I don't think it's so important what you think when you train as it is to just get on with it and do it. I don't try to think about anything in particular. I am just careful not to get distracted." After his workouts, however, Frank makes notes in his training log and reviews his training session in his mind. At that point, if he sees some room for

improvement, he makes a mental note.

One area involving visualization that many coaches agree can be helpful is overcoming weight, speed and distance barriers. For instance, if a bodybuilder is trying to squat or press a certain weight that is difficult, he could visualize a pair of hands reaching out to help him lift the weight. A runner might see in his mind a rope stretching ahead toward the finishing line and reeling him toward it. Lou Ferrigno used to visualize pictures of Arnold as he trained to beat him in the Mr. Olympia contest. The emotion of that image inspired him to greater efforts.

One area where all bodybuilders could profit from mental imagery techniques is in the preparation for competition. The presentation of the physique on stage, the movement, the posing—all can be aided by mental rehearsal. As the mind goes, so goes the body, and many a defeat can be traced to a bodybuilder having imagined the worst instead of developing a positive mental outlook.

"I go over my entire presentation in my mind," admits Zane. "Sometimes, when I have an exhibition to do and very little time to prepare, I rehearse my posing routine thoroughly in my mind until I can visualize it perfectly. This is especially valuable when I am making changes in the routine and don't have much time to really practice them."

Guided imagery, visualization and other mind power techniques are being increasingly explored both in and out of sports. They are becoming a factor in so-called "holistic" medicine. Christian Scientists have likely been using them a long time. The changing of self-image is useful in everything from gaining confidence in your social life to losing weight. But what is useful to some people is of paramount importance to bodybuilders.

The only way to achieve greatness in bodybuilding is to go beyond what you've ever done before, or ever believed possible. Before you crash through those physical barriers, you must believe you can. The extra effort derived from this is critical to your own achievements. It is not enough to just want to, no matter how desperately, unless you can translate this desire into effort.

Summoning the power of the mind through these new techniques combines the power of mind and body. It can lift you to new heights in bodybuilding.

Bodybuilding Workouts:

How Often Is Best?

by Larry Scott

"If you work out every day, the muscles will constantly wear down. It's only while you are resting that you are building," I heard him say. Eagerly, I waited for another "pearl" of wisdom to drop from the lips of the gym hero. After all, I reasoned, he had been training for over two years and had placed in a physique contest.

It was in the Old American Health Studio on Hollywood Boulevard. I had just sold everything I had which could be used to raise cash in my delirium to head for the West Coast to become famous. Pocatello, Idaho, was too small for me and I was firmly planted in a small rooming house across from the Hollywood Ranch Market. The Hollywood Health Club was about 15 minutes by foot from my boarding house. Though my only means of transportation was sole leather, I was in heaven during each intense moment I spent pounding the weights in the studio overlooking Hollywood Boulevard.

Ben Truman was really feeling good about the rapt attention he was getting from two Idaho boys as he expansively displayed his "deep" knowledge of training insight.

It seems we can receive expert advice on any subject from almost any caliber of participant. I

suppose bodybuilding is certainly no exception. The question of how many days or times per week we should hit the iron has been discussed as much as any subject on training.

Recently, having decided to train for the Olympia, I decided to throw out my old notions of training and see if I could discover something I hadn't learned before. My first question was how many times per week should I train. Using the instinctive training concept as my guide, I embarked on the following journey:

First, I reasoned, why not use the three-day system and see if I could make gains on it? This system meant I had to work the entire body each workout and repeat it three times per week. I knew, without even trying it, that I would be dead in a week. I believe that intensity of effort is extremely important in each workout, but the nature of my physique is such that I must do at least 10 sets to work up to total intensity.

I knew that physiologically I could not endure the battle of working without coasting at the beginning or the end of the workout, and so I decided that three-day-a-week workouts are definitely out for me. I don't have the energy or the willpower to totally blast each muscle group

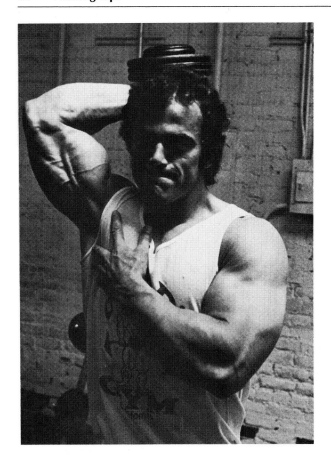

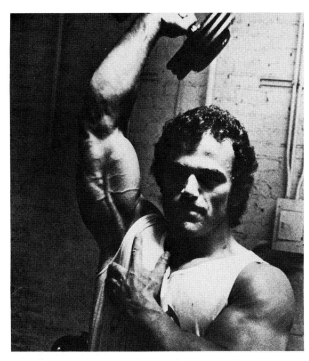

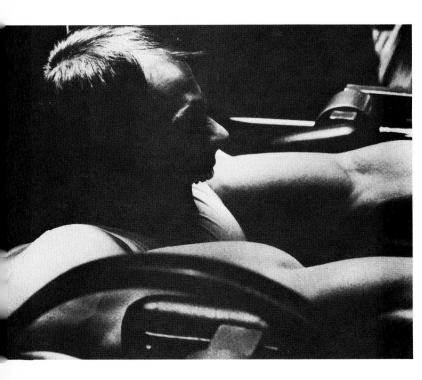

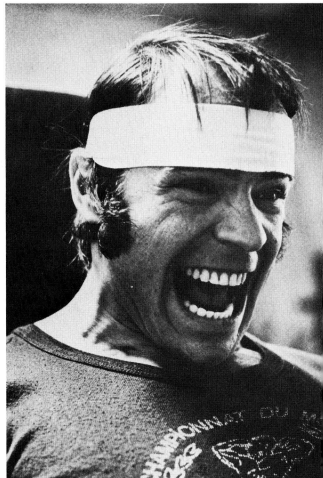

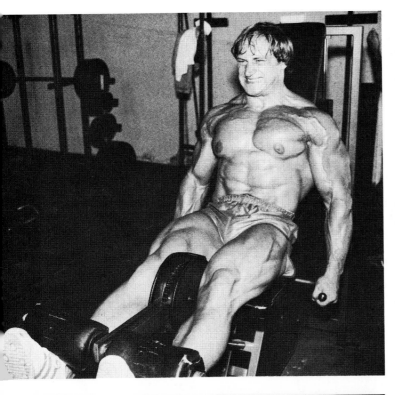

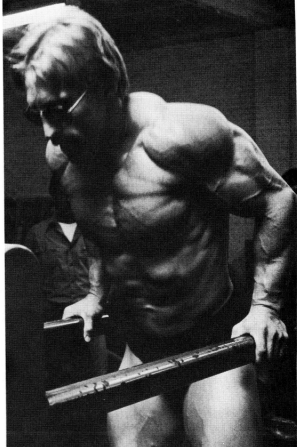

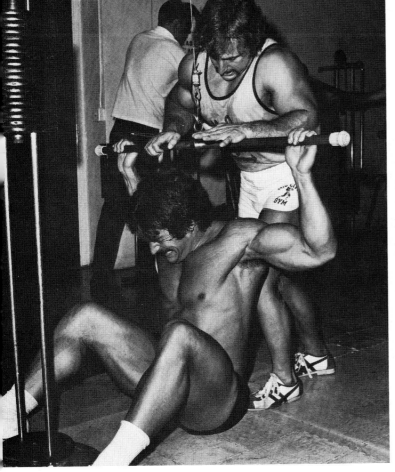

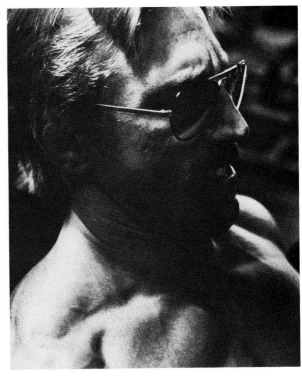

each workout. I don't care if I rested a week, I still couldn't put enough into each muscle group. Besides, I want my workout to be fun, not nauseating.

If the three-days-per-week workout won't work, how about the four-days-a-week system? This would involve doing the Weider Split System four times weekly. The body is still being worked twice per week, but the workout is now divided in half. How should one divide the workout?

Monday and Thursday should be pecs, lats, thighs and abs. Tuesday and Friday should be delts, arms, calves and forearms. Not a bad split, actually. I only see a few compromises. The first and most obvious is the fact that one has to work three major muscle groups and a minor one in one night. It's hard to sustain the intensity even with this system of split. Another problem is working the forearms on the same night as arms. It's a bad combination but to switch forearms and abs around is even worse.

Another problem with the four-day system is the long rest each week. Three days of rest is too much for an advanced trainer. In summary, the four-days-a-week system would be best for an intermediate bodybuilder or a dedicated beginner. It is also designed for those working with moderate intensity.

The next system would be the five-days-a-week program. This requires one to approach workouts on a continuing basis rather than by the week. This split is the same as a six-day split except you only work out five days per week. This requires borrowing one day from the next week to get through the entire body twice. The split would be as follows:

Monday
  Delts, Arms, Neck

Tuesday
  Thighs, Calves, Abs

Wednesday
  Pecs, Lats, Forearms

Thursday
  Delts, Arms, Neck

Friday
  Thighs, Calves, Abs

Monday
  Pecs, Lats, Forearms

This is an excellent split system which works well for the fellow who can't get to the gym on weekends. There are almost no compromises in this program except for the long rest over the weekend. Also, I have grouped the muscles together, which is popular today.

Then, of course, we have the six-day training program—same as the five-day workout except

Saturday is used, rather than spilling over into the next week to complete the double series.

Here's how I utilize the Weider Double Split system. This program is for advanced trainers and is generally used before a contest. It requires excellent nutrition and doubling up on all your supplements. You will really learn something about yourself while you are on this program.

The Double Split requires working out twice a day, five days per week. It's excellent for cutting up and hammering home a slow or stubborn body part. I must caution you, however—it's not for the beginner and it's not something you could endure for months at a time.

The Monday morning workout should be your high attention workout. Pick the body parts which are slow, stubborn or just need an extra shot to get peaked. A typical five-day double split would be:

Monday am
  Pecs, Thighs, Abs

Monday pm
  Lats, Arms, Neck

Tuesday am
  Delts, Calves, Forearms

Tuesday pm
  Pecs, Thighs, Abs

Wednesday am
  Lats, Arms, Neck

Wednesday pm
  Delts, Calves, Forearms

Thursday am
  Pecs, Thighs, Abs

Thursday pm
  Lats, Arms, Neck

Friday am
  Delts, Calves, Forearms

Friday pm
  Pecs, Thighs, Abs

Notice that the Monday morning workout is repeated four times. The others are done three times.

The disadvantage of this program is the super drain of energy. The intensity of the workouts suffer. Also, for many, the morning workout is tough to get started. It seems the joints are stiff. You're not fully awake, but you'll feel great when it's over. The psychological trauma of exerting so much willpower during the week will eventually cut into your stamina, but the weekends will become deliciously relaxing.

Remember, my views are purely a matter of trial and error. I have experimented with each one of the programs which I have discussed. The result is purely my subjective opinion. Take it for what it's worth.

Based upon your own physical limitations, you will begin to design your workouts with different intensity factors for different muscle groups. For example, if your thighs respond well to training but your calves are slow and stubborn, you will find yourself spending more time and intensity on your slower areas.

It is with that thought in mind, as well as the natural symmetry of the body, that I proceed with a brief explanation of anti-stress grouping. Deltoids and arms, for me, are both extremely hard workouts so I don't want to do them on the same night. Yet I need something to warm up my arms, so they must be done second. The lat workout is excellent for warming up the elbows and lower biceps connector, so I combine lats, arms, and neck on the same night. That leaves delts, thighs, calves, forearms and abs.

Deltoids are hard and nothing will really warm up the shoulders except light shoulder work, so I do them first when I'm full of energy. I could combine calves with deltoids, but after I'm through with delts, I'm a little tired and I have fought the pain quite well. The battle with calves and the extreme pain associated with them may not go well with delts.

I find myself withdrawing a little from the pain of high reps on calf raises if I have already drained a lot of my pain reserve while doing dumbbell presses, heavy dumbbell laterals and bent-over laterals. For me, the combination of delts and thighs works best. Thighs are hard but the reps are short and I like the exhaustion of heavy thigh work better than the long agony of calf work; so I combine delts, thighs and forearms.

That leaves pecs, calves and abdominals, which act like members of the same family. Pecs are low pain, calves are high pain and abdominals are not compromised with arms. That seems to be one of the best anti-stress groups I have come up with; but, as always, it is constantly changing and a month from now I'm sure something will be different. Hope you can use the ideas.

A brief explanation of the Weider Instinctive Training Principle: My body tells me what is good rather than my brain telling my body. I personally have found more success with this system than any other I have been able to devise or copy.

The Thinking Man's Repetition

by Casey Viator

I doubt that any exercise of any consequence remains undiscovered. So rather than looking for new exercises, we should more fully explore the dynamics of a series of repetitions, better known as a set.

Until the bodybuilder has learned how to apply the proper force to every repetition, he will never get the mass and cuts he seeks. People often ask me for a new exercise for this or that body part. I advise them to learn how to properly perform the exercises they already know.

There is a great deal more to an exercise than just going through X number of reps for X number of sets. Without the full realization of the biodynamics of a set of reps, your muscles quickly adapt to habit patterns that result in exasperating impasses.

Whether an exercise is going to build the muscle you want or leave you stranded with a persistent lack of progress is determined by four main points which we'll cover below. A beginner should learn these immediately and the veteran would do well to review them.

1. *Speed of Repetition*—If you're using the correct weight in an exercise, you should be able

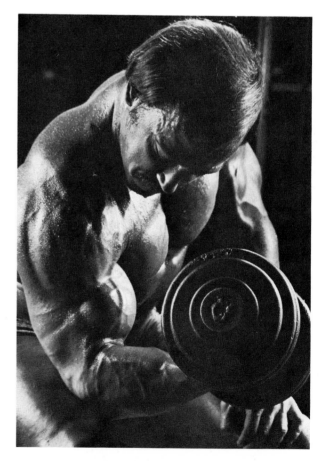

Carve out a spot for yourself among bodybuilding's elite with this intelligent, progressive approach to training.

to perform the first seven reps in rather strict form—three seconds for concentric contraction (raising the weight), two seconds for eccentric contraction (lowering the weight). In other words, a repetition from full flexion to full extension should take five seconds.

As successive reps grow harder, there is a tendency to speed up the movement. If greater speed is required before the seventh rep, it means the weight is probably too heavy. The first seven reps should be of uniform speed.

After the seventh rep, you should try to speed up the movement. Notice I said "try." After pre-fatiguing the muscle with strict reps, it's difficult to do more reps without cheating, using other muscles to gain momentum. If, instead of cheating the movement, you make an effort to speed it up, you will find that the remaining five reps (for a total of 12 reps) can be done in the same strict form as the initial reps.

After the 10th rep, a tingling numbness occurs. That's the time the muscle is firing the deeper fibers. The outer fibers have already been exhausted, and the deeper fibers are mobilized to take their place. That's when muscle growth really begins to occur.

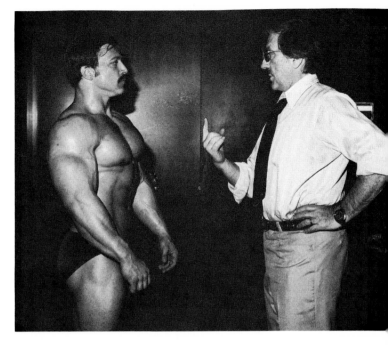

"During my regular visits to Weider headquarters, Joe always advises me on my training and posing."

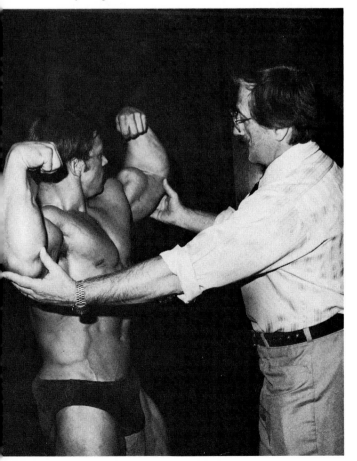

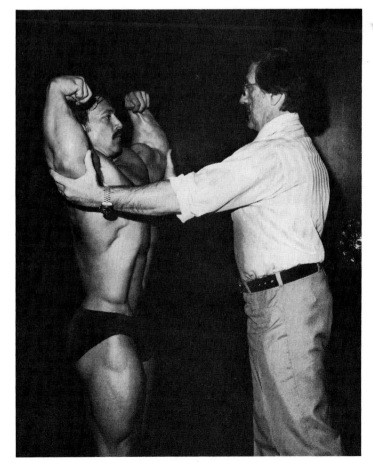

It's possible to dig even a bit further into a given muscle group by pre-exhausting the muscle with an indirect exercise beforehand. For example, do a set of Close-Grip Chins and proceed immediately to a heavy set of Barbell Curls, taking no rest between the two sets. The first exercise is a primer for the second.

It is necessary to exert maximum power in order to stimulate growth, but it's not important to exert this power during the first part of a set of reps. Maximum power should be applied starting at about the seventh rep and continued to the twelfth rep. By the seventh rep you hit pay dirt, and you continue digging.

This approach serves a dual purpose. First, it gives you maximum results. Second, it offers insurance against injury. By speeding up the final reps, you intensify your concentration and your body automatically marshalls a heavy reserve of muscle to execute the additional reps. Remember, you only get hurt when you are not concentrating.

2. *Positive/Negative Set*—When you finally get the feel of doing a regular set, in the above manner, you can expand on the concept by adding negative reps. The assistance of a training partner is needed, although some dumbbell negative reps can be performed without a partner.

At the end of a positive set of 12 reps in which you have worked to failure, additional reps can be performed by having a training partner assist you in raising the weight so you can then lower the weight by yourself. Lower the weight slowly for a count of eight seconds. As you continue these negative reps, the muscle (or muscle group) will become weaker, and the weight will naturally drop faster. When you can no longer control the movement, stop!

Negative reps will fire even deeper muscle fibers than you are able to involve in the positive part of the set. You have literally crossed the threshold of your emergency reserve, an area reserved for fight-or-flight conditions. You are literally building muscle to save your life.

However, negative reps should be done only twice a week. Overtraining is a constant threat when you're doing this type of training, so you must proceed with caution.

3. *Progressive Set*—It's hard for the beginner to appreciate the degree of effort put forth by the top bodybuilders. The big guys live according to a tenet of *progressive resistance*. The longer this resistance is applied, the bigger and stronger their muscles become. Maximum

muscle growth can only be achieved by expanding your sets every workout through the addition of weights or repetitions.

Strict written records should be maintained to guarantee that your workouts are progressively harder. Your training partner can count and record your reps and sets, and you can reciprocate. Without a written record, it's almost impossible to remember how many reps and sets

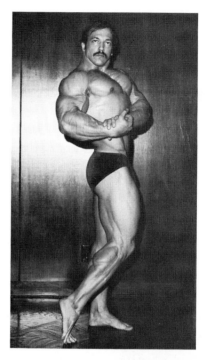

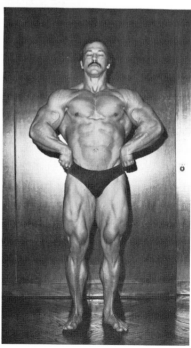

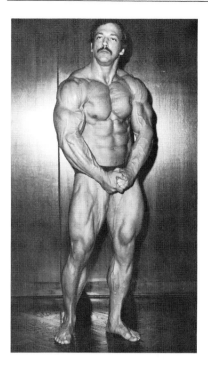

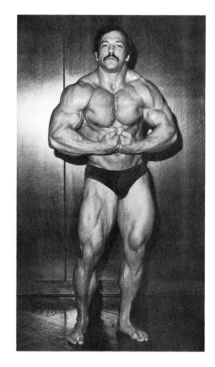

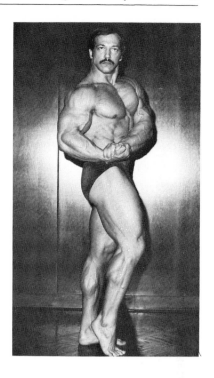

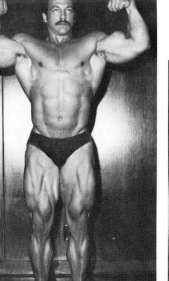

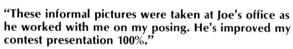

"These informal pictures were taken at Joe's office as he worked with me on my posing. He's improved my contest presentation 100%."

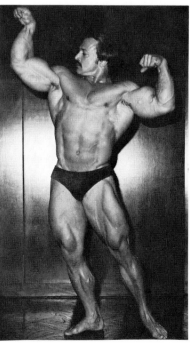

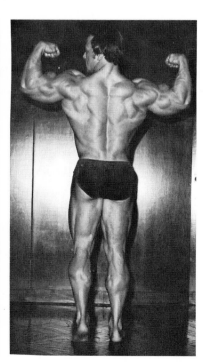

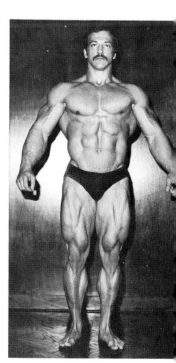

you did in a given exercise in a previous workout.

By keeping careful written records, you can make comparisons on a seasonal or yearly basis that actually allows you to predict future gains or make better adjustments. This is a great boon to the competitive bodybuilder.

4. *Repetition Count*—Whenever you can perform 15 reps with a given weight for any lower body exercise, it's time to increase the weight in the next workout. Add enough weight so that you'll only be able to do 10-12 strict positive reps. You might stay at the new weight for a couple of workouts, during which time your reps will climb back up to 15. Again, add weight in the subsequent workout.

When you can perform 12 reps with a given weight for any *upper* body exercise, increase the weight in the next workout, but do not add so much weight that you fall below 10 reps.

You probably shouldn't do more than two sets on a particular exercise. After doing two sets, it's better to move on to a new exercise, hitting the same body part from a different angle. You won't need to do more than four different exercises per body part if you follow the system that has been outlined: Speed of Repetition, Positive/Negative Set, Progressive Set and Repetition Count.

I have personally used this system throughout my bodybuilding career. It has helped put me in the top echelon of competitors. By using this system, you can make room at the top for yourself, too.

Updating High-Intensity Methods

by Mike Mentzer

"One of the world's greatest and most scientific bodybuilders, Mike Mentzer, brings *Muscle & Fitness* readers more interesting and helpful information with this detailed report on high-intensity training. I assigned Mike the task of doing this report so that our readers could share in his broad awareness of the science of bodybuilding."—Joe Weider

It's fairly obvious that to build big muscles and increase your strength, you must lift weights. But the number of letters I get from bodybuilders asking me how they can build bigger arms, rounder pecs, thicker delts, etc., shows that what isn't so obvious is *how* to lift weights and *what kinds* of workouts one should do to build big muscles.

Those who read two of my articles in *Muscle & Fitness*—"Up the Ladder of Intensity," (Oct. 1979 issue) and "Raising Your Muscle Building Consciousness," (July 1980 issue)—hopefully gained more insight into this question of how to train. In these articles I stressed that only by generating progressively stronger muscular contractions do we build muscle tissue. I also offered hints on how to generate such contraction.

What remains obscure to so many

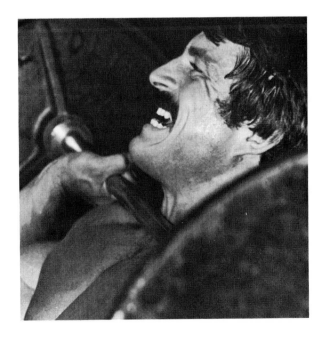

bodybuilders, as evidenced by the many questions I receive in letters and at public appearances, is how to progressively increase the intensity of muscular contraction. This obscurity arises in part from the fact that many still do not fully understand the concept of intensity.

"Intensity" is a term that has been bandied about a lot lately in all the bodybuilding periodicals. Very rarely, however, is intensity described accurately. It's obvious when reading the various articles that the authors—including certain top bodybuilders—still confuse intensity with duration. Apparently the authors in these cases have not grasped the fundamental relationship that exists between the two.

Intensity and duration are, for one thing, mutually exclusive. Only when a muscle is contracting with the greatest possible force at any given moment is there maximum intensity. When you're training in such a way that every rep of every set of every exercise requires an absolute maximum effort, the duration of that workout must be and will be brief. High-intensity muscular contraction, in other words, prevents a large number of such contractions.

So maximum training intensity limits the duration of your training. What's even more significant is that anything less than maximum intensity will result in less than optimal results.

A wise, old man once likened exercise and muscle growth to a stick of dynamite and a hammer. Hitting a stick of dynamite lightly with a hammer will not produce an explosion no matter how many times you hit it. If, however, you hit it very hard, only one blow is required to stimulate or produce an explosion.

Much the same situation exists in stimulating growth with weight training. No amount of light or low-intensity training will produce an increase. High-intensity training is a basic requirement in producing the desired physical change. Large quantities of such stimulation are not necessary, nor are they desired. In other words, it takes only one hard blow from the hammer to set off the explosion of the dynamite.

Personal experience has taught most of us that high-intensity training produces an effect on our bodies that we never get from low-intensity work. The effect that training of different intensity levels has upon our systems can be better understood if we look at an intensity continuum (see below) in which complete inactivity and rest constitute one extreme and absolute, all-out effort constitutes the other. The effect each extreme has on our system is obviously very different.

These are just four indices registering the change in our systems when we go from a state of rest to one of all-out effort. Of course, there are many more indices, such as pH and lactic acid levels, but you get the idea.

High-intensity training is hard training, and as such, it has a definite effect on our systems. This effect can be measured in the lab and felt subjectively by the individual doing the training.

The effect is dramatic and can be very uncomfortable. Whereas rest and total inactivity are experienced as comfortable, training at maximum intensity is brutal and uncomfortable. If you are able to talk between sets and feel the desire to add more sets to your workouts, then you're not training with maximum intensity. If you are training with maximum effort, you won't be able to talk between sets because you'll be breathing too hard. And instead of thinking about more sets, you'll begin looking for excuses to *shorten* your workouts.

While intensity is necessary for anyone wishing to build muscle, and its effects are similar on everyone, intensity remains a relative measure, contingent upon an individual's existing level of strength and development. Let's face it, a 12-inch

Rest—Total Inactivity (lowest possible intensity)	Maximum Effort (highest possible intensity)
Pulse rate: slow—60–75 beats per minute	Pulse rate: fast—150–220 beats per minute
Breathing: shallow and slow—12–14 breaths per minute	Breathing: very rapid—50–100 breaths per minute
O_2 Uptake (ventilation-oxygen uptake ratio): 20–25	O_2 Uptake: 30
Respiratory Exchange Index (Energy exchange within body—partial measure of body metabolism): 0.825	Respiratory Exchange Index: 1.20

arm contracting maximally will not require the same amount of fuel or produce the same quantities of by-products and wastes as a 20-inch arm contracting maximally. Since we require increasingly greater contractions if we hope to continually progress, we must search for increasingly brutal methods to provide such contractions as we get stronger. For the beginner, just about any form of resistance exercise will represent an increase in intensity to his overall system. As he progresses to the intermediate and advanced stage, however, he will require increasingly intense training methods.

Below I have outlined the essentials of weight-resistence exercise that apply to everyone regardless of existing development. Also, I have provided a breakdown of various intensity methods for beginners, intermediates and advanced bodybuilders.

ESSENTIALS OF WEIGHT-RESISTANCE EXERCISE

As a first step in learning *how* to lift weights for bigger and stronger muscles, we must understand the essential components involved. When we lift a barbell, we aren't just lifting a certain amount of weight; we are lifting that weight over a certain distance in a certain amount of time. The three factors (or essential components) are weight, distance and time. If we wish to increase our individual training intensity, we must cause our muscles to generate more horsepower. This is done by lifting heavier weights over greater distances in shorter periods of time.

Adjusting the amount of weight we lift in any particular exercise is the easiest factor to understand and apply to our workouts. Whenever there is an increase in strength, the amount of weight used in that exercise should be increased. If you can currently bench press 250 pounds for six maximum repetitions, and two weeks from now you can bench press the same weight for 10 maximum reps, the weight should be increased by approximately 5-10%, or whatever amount is required to lower your maximum rep performance to six once again. Still later, when you can do 10 reps with the heavier weight, increase the poundage another 5-10%. Keep increasing the weight as you increase your strength. Such is the nature of progressive weight-resistance exercise.

Since the lengths of our bones are fixed, there isn't much we can do to increase the distance over which we move the weights in most of our exercises. The distance you move a weight in the Barbell Curl, for instance, is directly related to the length of your forearms. And unless you are young and still growing, that distance, for all intents and purposes, will remain fixed and unalterable.

Lifting weights in shorter periods of time is a relatively simple matter but subject to some misunderstanding. In speaking of the speed on a isolated repetition, the weight should be moved from a position of full extension to one of full contraction in the shortest possible time, utilizing only the force of muscular contraction.

In reality, this turns out to be a relatively slow movement, especially if the weight is heavy. When the speed exceeds a certain rate, momentum takes over and is responsible for completing the movement. And remember that intensity refers to muscular contraction. Momentum is an outside force which will diminish intensity if you're not careful. All your exercises, therefore, should be initiated deliberately, with no sudden thrusts or jerks, and carried to completion relatively slowly, with the weight always under control.

When referring to the amount of time between sets, only rest long enough so you can resume with enough efficiency to carry the next set to muscular failure. If rest time is too brief, your next set will terminate at a point of cardiovascular failure instead of muscular failure. And if the rest is too long, the muscle will cool off, preventing maximum effort.

To summarize, therefore, the amount of weight lifted, the amount of time it takes to lift the weight, and the rest time between sets determines intensity. Distance will be a fixed value, not subject to adjustment (at least on conventional equipment). The following methods are based on these simple features and, if followed correctly, they will definitely enhance your progress.

TRAINING TO FAILURE

Putting aside all academic and theoretical considerations for a moment, what we are talking about here, quite simply, is hard work—gut-busting, all-out effort! Any degree of effort below maximum may yield the bodybuilder some results but never on the same order as all-out effort. And, again, when I say "all-out effort," I'm not referring to the performance of marathon workouts involving set after set after set until you fall over from fatique.

Training to a point of momentary muscular failure, where the completion of another full rep is impossible despite your greatest effort, is the only way to force the body to resort to its reserves sufficiently to stimulate real growth. None of us needs to be reminded that growth never comes easy; it must literally be forced!

Ending a set just because an arbitrary number of reps has been completed will do little or nothing to stimulate growth. If you can curl 100 pounds for 10 reps and you never try to do that 11th rep, your body has no reason to alter itself, to grow. The body will always attempt to maintain the existing situation. Only when you impose some extraordinary demand upon it will it change. You needn't be a physiologist to understand that.

Carrying a set to a point of momentary muscular failure ensures that you pass through the "break-over" point—the level of effort in the set at which growth stimulation commences. Where is that point? Is it at 85% of maximum effort? Is it at 90%? No one knows for sure, but you can be certain that if you train at 100% effort, you will have reached the "break-over" point.

For those who are just taking up weight training, I suggest you proceed with caution at first. If you have been sedentary most of your life, weight training will represent a radical departure for you. Training to absolute failure may not only be unnecessary but dangerous. The first several months should be spent learning proper exercise form and developing a sense of your capacities.

As you develop confidence in handling weights and you gain added muscle and strength, start carrying each and every set (not including warm-up sets) to a point of momentary muscular failure. Select a weight in each exercise that will allow approximately six reps in strict form. Maximum reps in strict form means going to a point where you can no longer raise the weight in perfectly strict fashion from a point of complete extension to one of full contraction. This method of training to failure should be followed by everyone wishing to induce maximum muscle growth.

PRE-FATIGUE

As mentioned above, it's imperative that we pass through the "break-over" point in intensity by carrying each set to a point of momentary failure. This is impossible, however, on exercises involving two or more muscles when one of these is a so-called weak link.

Most conventional weight exercises for the chest, for example, involve the triceps. The triceps, being a smaller and, therefore, weaker muscle, will prevent you from working the pectorals to a point of failure. If you can incline 200 pounds for six reps, it's not the pectorals that are preventing you from lifting more weight or doing more reps. It's the weaker triceps giving out first.

A similar situation exists when we work the lats with conventional rowing, chinning or pulldown movements. The biceps are unavoidably involved in these exercises because the upper arms must bend. Since the biceps are smaller and weaker than the much larger latissimus muscles, they will give out first, preventing the lats from being worked to the maximum and receiving full growth stimulation.

This situation can be remedied by first performing an exercise that isolates and tires the primary muscle group. For example, Cable Crossovers, Dumbbell Flyes and Nautilus Flyes serve to isolate the pecs. By carrying one of these exercises to a point of failure and then proceeding immediately to an exercise that involves the pecs along with a secondary muscle—say, the triceps, in the case of the chest—the triceps will have a temporary strength advantage over the "pre-fatigued" pectoral muscles. This will serve to enhance your chest work, rather than hinder it.

This will only be the case, however, as long as there is zero rest between the first isolation exercise and the second compound exercise (a compound exercise is one in which more than one muscle group is used to move the resistance). Taking any more rest than the time it takes to move from one piece of equipment to the other will seriously compromise the effectiveness of this method as the pre-fatigued muscle will regain up to 50% of its strength within 3-5 seconds of completion of the set!

Examples of pre-fatigue exercise sequences follow:
Pecs—
   1. Flyes
   2. Bench Press
   1. Cable Crossovers
   2. Dips
   1. Pec Deck
   2. Incline Presses
Lats—
   1. Dumbbell Pullover
   2. Barbell Row

1. Nautilus Pullover
2. Chins (palms up)
1. Straight-Arm Pulldown
2. Regular Pulldown (palms up)

Delts—
   1. Dumbbell Laterals
   2. Press Behind Neck
   1. Nautilus Laterals
   2. Nautilus Press

Traps—
   1. Shrugs (barbell, dumbbell, Nautilus)
   2. Upright Rows

Thighs—
   1. Leg Extensions
   2. Leg Press or Squat

Triceps—
   1. Pressdowns
   2. Dips
   1. French Press
   2. Close-Grip Bench Press

Biceps—
   1. Barbell Curls
   2. Close-Grip, Palms-Up Pulldown
   1. Nautilus Curls
   2. Palms-Up Chins

NOTE: *In training the triceps and biceps, the pecs and lats aren't weak links. But compound exercises involving the latter two muscles can help the triceps and biceps continue working after being fatigued by an isolation exercise.*

TIPS ON USING PRE-FATIGUE

1. Keep the reps fairly low in a pre-fatigue superset since you are doing two consecutive sets. Too many reps—more than 10—can lead to labored breathing, and could prevent you from continuing the exercise until muscular failure is reached. Six strict reps is best.

2. Never perform more than two pre-fatigue cycles or supersets.

3. Beginners don't necessarily require pre-fatigue. Intermediates and advanced bodybuilders can add forced reps and negatives to either one or both of the exercises in the pre-fatigue cycle.

4. Don't get stuck on using pre-fatigue, or any other method, exclusively. Using pre-fatigue once a week for each body part is sufficient.

PEAK CONTRACTION

If you read my series of articles on the various Weider principles, you'll recall that I referred to the Peak Contraction Principle as perhaps the most important.

As I've already stated in this article, we must generate progressively stronger muscular contractions to stimulate maximum increases in size and strength. In order to assure maximum contractions, two conditions must be met: 1) Since muscle fibers contract by reducing their length, a muscle would have to be in the fully contracted, or peak, position if all the fibers were to be contracted simultaneously; 2) And to get all the fibers contracted at the same time, one would have to impose a load that was intense enough to activate all of the muscle's fibers.

When a muscle moves against a heavy resistance through a full range of motion (i.e., from a position of full extension to one of complete contraction), more and more fibers come into play until peak contraction is reached. At peak contraction, no further movement is possible and the maximum number of fibers have been activated. The Weider Peak Contraction Principle comes into play in those exercises which provide resistance in the peak contraction position, the most important point in the range of motion of any exercise.

In choosing the best exercises for peak contraction, select those that make you "fight" to hold the weight at the top. The regular Barbell Curl is a poor exercise (unless it's angled) because once you pass mid-range, effective resistance falls off dramatically. Exercises such as Leg Extensions, Triceps Pressdowns, Chins and various Nautilus movements provide resistance in the contracted position, allowing for higher intensity of contraction when sufficient weight is handled. When formulating a routine, select at least one exercise for each body part that involves this important Weider Principle.

FORCED REPS

Anything you do to make your training harder—not longer, but more brutal moment to moment—will raise the intensity and the effectiveness of your workouts. After you've reached a point of failure where another strict rep is impossible despite the greatest effort, you can increase the intensity still more by having your training partner assist you in the completion of two or three forced reps. In most cases, it's best to keep the same weight on the bar and have your partner assist you just enough so that you can barely complete the rep with all-out, gut-busting effort.

Many people write me asking if reducing the

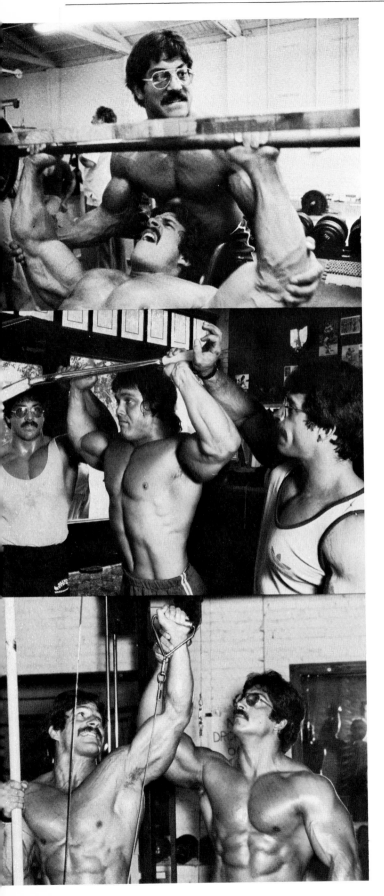

weight and completing several more reps is just as good. The answer is "no." If you reduce the weight too much, the next rep will not require maximum, all-out effort. So the intensity actually will fall below the level of the last strict rep you completed on your own. Keeping the weight the same and getting just enough assistance from a partner who is in tune with you assures an increase in intensity.

Forced reps aren't necessary for beginners for reasons already discussed. Intermediates might add forced reps to one of the exercises in the pre-fatigue sequence, either the isolation exercise or the compound movement. Advanced bodybuilders probably would do well to try forced reps on both the isolation and compound exercises of that sequence.

I wouldn't recommend doing forced reps every workout necessarily, especially for intermediates. Intermediates should take each body part to positive failure in one workout, to positive failure with forced reps the next workout, and to negative failure in the third workout.

The advanced bodybuilder who requires higher intensity and is more in tune with his physical needs (Weider Instinctive Principle) should play it by ear. An advanced man may want to depart from the suggested rep protocol of six strict positive reps followed by forced reps. Since his larger and stronger muscles place much greater demands on his cardio-respiratory and other physical systems during very heavy contraction, he may want to use weights that only allow a maximum of four strict positive reps. It's a matter of using one's judgment.

NEGATIVE REPS
(THE WEIDER REVERSE GRAVITY PRINCIPLE)

Our skeletal muscles possess three types of strength: 1) Positive strength, or the ability to raise a weight; 2) Static, or holding strength; 3) Negative strength, or our ability to lower a weight. We are weakest in positive strength and strongest in negative strength.

Obviously, we can't really say we've trained to failure until we've also exhausted our ability to lower the weight. Only by continuing to lower a weight after completing six positive reps and two forced reps—which will exhaust your positive

To totally crash the pain barrier, you need the help of a partner or two.

and static strength levels—can you reach a point of true and absolute momentary muscular failure.

Having completed your six positives and two forced reps, have your partner, or partners, lift the weight to the top (or peak contracted position) so that you can lower it. You'll probably be surprised at your ability to continue lowering a weight even after you've reached positive failure.

The first few negatives will seem very easy and you'll be able to lower the weight slowly. The next couple of reps will become difficult, however. The downward movement will pick up speed, and you won't have as much control. End the set when you can no longer control the descent of the weight, or stop a rep prior to that, as a heavy weight yanking a body part out of the contracted position can be dangerous.

On certain exercises involving large and powerful muscles, like the thighs, be very careful. I would advise against doing Squats in this manner for obvious safety reasons, and even Thigh Extensions can be dangerous.

You may find that the weight you used for six positive reps will be too light for continued negatives. If that's the case, your partner will have to apply manual resistance as you lower the weight. Do not, I repeat, *do not* attempt to halt the downward motion of the weight when you're doing negatives. The knees tend to be delicate. If you fight against a maximum negative resistance, you could cause severe injury to the knees.

Beginners don't require negatives as it is a high-intensity method reserved for ambitious intermediates and advanced bodybuilders. Negatives also can be done in a "pure" style— i.e., they don't have to be preceded by positive and forced reps. Take a weight that's at least 40% heavier than you would normally use in positive fashion, have spotters raise it for you, and continue lowering the weight slowly until you're beginning to lose control. Make sure your spotters remain alert to what you're doing so they can grab the weight as soon as you signal for them to do so.

Entire workouts can be done in this fashion or combined with positive and forced reps as described earlier. Be innovative and improvise. The isolation portion of the pre-fatigue superset can be done positive/forced/negative fashion and the compound exercise of the same superset in negative style only, for example.

There are limitless combinations and ways of employing all these methods so that no two workouts need be the same. I would advise against using negatives in every workout. Since the intensity is so high, it could lead to overtraining.

REST-PAUSE

Ever since first writing about rest-pause training back in the June 1979 issue of *Muscle Builder* (now *Muscle & Fitness*), I've been deluged with questions from bodybuilders wanting more information about it. The reason I haven't written about it since was that I trained for several contests this past year and rest-pause wasn't part of that preparation. Now, however, with the off-season upon us, I plan to get back to it and a few other Heavy Duty methods with a vengeance. With super-monster Casey Viator having made the move to California to train with me in high-intensity style, I should have some interesting things to report. The action at Gold's Gym is already getting so hot, with Casey and me tearing things up, that co-owner Pete Grymkowski has decided to take out fire insurance!

For those of you who don't have access to that first article I wrote on rest-pause, let me give you a quick review. As we climb steadily up the ladder of intensity, the demand for more brutal workouts increases. The problem for the advanced bodybuilder is compounded by mitigating physiological changes that accompany high growth and strength increases. A large and strong muscle contracting intensely and consecutively creates a profound oxygen debt and waste product buildup. As a matter of fact, total oxygen uptake in a muscle working at maximum capacity may increase 30 times! Muscle contractions can, however, become so intense that blood flow—and hence oxygen delivery—is decreased. In effect then, more time has to be allowed between contractions, or reps, for the vascular system to fill before the next contraction; thus, the concept of rest-pause training.

Further scientific evidence backing up the basis for rest-pause training can be found in the fine exercise physiology textbook by Edington and Edgerton entitled, *The Biology of Physical Exercise*. As stated in the book, "Blood flow to working muscles does not increase at high work intensities *when the duration of contractions is short enough, and the duration of relaxation is long enough."*

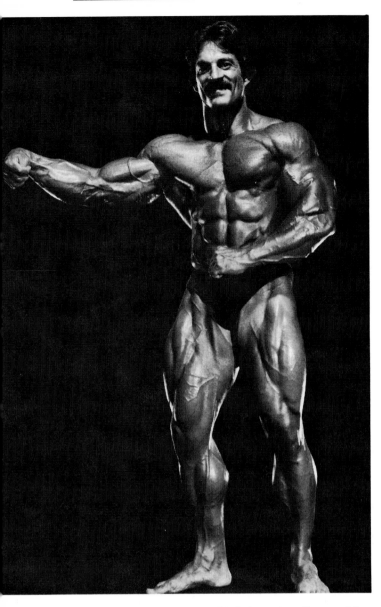

Only gut-busting, all-out, high-intensity effort could have built the herculean body of Mike Mentzer, one of the world's most massively developed men.

The bodybuilder can overcome the diminished capacity for continued high-intensity contraction by resting up to 10 seconds between reps. This rest-pause will allow blood to bring fuel to the working muscle, as well as rid the muscle of the metabolic by-products.

My use of this method involved the selection of a weight that allowed for one maximum rep in a particular exercise. After performing that one rep, I'd put the weight down, rest for 10 seconds and then do another rep. Usually by the second or third rep, I'd have to reduce the weight by 10% or have my partner provide just enough assistance to allow another maximum effort.

I would do one set of four reps for each exercise. Never did I do more than three total sets per body part. I experimented at first by resting 15 seconds between reps. Other times I rested for seven seconds. Fifteen turned out to be too long and seven seconds too short.

I also tried six reps per set, but I found it too taxing and it immediately led to overtraining. Doing four reps, with the 10-second rest-pause, I increased every single exercise at least 20 pounds per workout until I finally had improved 66% on each one. My size, of course, increased also.

Beginners and intermediates should save this training method for later in their bodybuilding careers when they need it. Advanced bodybuilders might want to experiment a bit with rest times and number of reps as I did. Keep in mind, however, that this is one of the most intense and brutal methods of training ever devised! Keep your sets low, and if progress is not immediately and dramatically forthcoming, you have exceeded your body's ability to cope with this intense form of stress—i.e., you're overtraining. You must realize that unlike the other methods of training where you perform one maximum effort per set, in rest-pause training every rep is maximum. While such effort is highly productive, it is also very, very taxing. BEWARE!

So there you have an update of high-intensity training methods. This discussion, of course, was not definitive and will continue in later issues of *Muscle & Fitness* as my investigations yield more interesting data for the Weider Research Clinic. Until then, train hard and good luck!

Secrets of Getting Ripped

by Tom Platz

It's never been particularly easy for me to rip up prior to a contest, and only through years of experience have I been able to come up with a personal formula that consistently works. This formula consists of proper combinations of training, nutrition and sun, plus a few other miscellaneous factors. In this article, I will explore each of these topics in detail, but first I want to comment on the relevance of the Weider Instinctive Training Principle to precontest training.

Everything I say in this article will concern what works for me, what I've found to work after many experiments. This does not necessarily mean that the techniques will work for you. You will need to make experiments on your own body over a period of time, using your instinct to determine what will ultimately be best for you.

Only you can become an instinctive trainer for your own body, so learn to monitor all of your body's biofeedback and learn from what your muscles tell you. If they pump up and grow, you're on the right track. And if you get progressively cut up from what you are doing prior to a contest, you are also on the right path.

So, as I unfold my four-pronged attack of

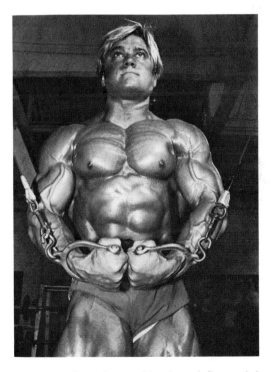

"Without the right combination of diet, training and sun, I'd never be able to get as ripped as I was for the Universe."

precontest training—the sun, nutrition, training, and miscellaneous factors—keep in mind that I do so only so you can try my methods and ultimately determine if they work for you. This is the essence of the Weider Instinctive Training

Principle—finding out what works for you, and then sticking to it until something even better comes along.

SUN

One of the most important items for me to get ripped is taking in sun. Of course this makes the skin darker, and the body looks harder when tanned, but I also utilize sun for dehydration. In the sun, water is excreted and the skin becomes thinner and tighter. The skin becomes so tight that it actually begins to hug the muscles, and vascularity comes out to the point that the veins look like a map of the Los Angeles freeway system.

I first became aware of the importance of skin tone and color at the first Mr. International contest I attended a couple years ago. Roger Callard was competing and he'd slightly mistimed his peak. Despite not being in his absolute best condition, he totally glowed in the line-up. His skin color and texture, as well as the way he stood in the line-up, got him to the top of his class.

After watching the way Roger laid out in the sun on Venice Beach and noticing some of the things he used, I adopted parts of his system. The result has been very gratifying, and at this point I can truthfully say that my contest success is about 40 percent from the sun.

Another individual who is a product of good sun usage is Frank Zane. I talked to him, and he hardly even trains the last week before a contest. Instead, he stays out in the sun as much as possible and practices his posing and stage presentation. Prior to the last Olympia, Zane went to Palm Springs for several days and stayed out in the sun almost the whole time. He used the sun a lot to get ripped.

After many experiments, I've found that baby oil and iodine are the best things for my skin when tanning. This is any brand of baby oil and regular iodine, as long as it's the kind that turns red. The mixture is usually 12 ounces of oil to one-1½ bottles of iodine, and I use this several times during the period I'm out in the sun. Whenever my skin begins to dry out, I put on another coating of the oil and iodine.

My experiments have shown that the best way to get a tan is to lie at various angles to be sure that the coloring is even. Sometimes you'll find that your chest is darker than your shoulders, so you'll need to orient your body toward the sun to put more rays on your shoulders for awhile.

After awhile, you can begin to walk along the beach and still maintain an even tan, but be sure to keep it even. A spotty tan is almost useless, since it distracts the eye away from the muscles.

Before the Universe, I was taking as much sun as I could. If I could have had sun seven days a week I would have, but sometimes the sun isn't out, even here in California. I took so much that I sometimes got a little light-headed, at which times I would have to back up a little bit and take it easier. This probably comes from losing too much water one day, because I usually don't drink anything while in the sun. I'm never in the sun more than three hours, and the best time for me is usually between 11 am and 3 pm.

As with other contest preparation factors, sunning must be timed. If you start too early, you can hit your peak prematurely and stay dehydrated too long. It's extremely difficult to train that way, because it causes you to be lethargic. You have to develop the timing to know when to get a lot of sun and when not to get sun. This comes only through experimentation and experience.

DIET

It takes experimentation—with various amounts of trial and error—to arrive at the optimum personal formula of individual caloric consumption close to a contest. Factors like what kinds of calories and when they can be consumed also come into play, in addition to how many calories you consume.

In order to get cut, I have to stay hungry all day, and go to bed hungry at night. In the past, I didn't subscribe to the idea of staying away from food for several hours before bedtime, but this year I've tried that method and am a true believer. I would never eat anything closer than two hours before retiring. This year I experimented with eating more, but nothing close to bedtime, and still achieved the fat losses I wanted.

I eat four times a day before a contest. In the morning it's eggs, at mid-day red meat and for the last two meals tuna or chicken. Before the Universe I was consuming 3000–3300 calories and exactly 30 grams of carbohydrate per day. I'd eat my carbohydrates in the morning, usually in the form of canteloupe. In the evening I'd sometimes eat minor amounts of carbohydrate via lettuce, vinegar and tuna fish.

Every year I seem to get hooked on different fruits for the carbs. Once it was apples, then grapefruit, and now I don't think it matters what fruit you eat. Maybe bananas have a little too much sodium causing you to retain water, but otherwise no fruit will blur your definition if taken in small amounts. It will also provide training energy. I do like things you can eat a lot of and canteloupe is a large fruit with very little carbohydrate in relation to its size. It makes me feel good to eat a lot more. I've learned how to trick my mind to make it think I'm eating more than I actually am.

It's important to gradually reduce your carbs as the contest approaches. Toward the end, you're consuming just enough to train on, and that's it. I never go to zero anymore, because completely eliminating carbohydrates is a mistake. You have to have some carbs, or you will burn out and won't be able to get a pump when training. On the last day, I overload on carbohydrates.

Defining supplements are an individual thing. I can get cut without choline and inositol, although I do take as much as I can of both before a contest. I believe they help me to lose fat at a faster rate. The choline and inositol are also good for my health. And when you are training hard and dieting, it is important to take in calcium and other minerals. If your body runs low on calcium, you'll feel very jittery, and without enough minerals—particularly potassium—you will lack training energy.

TRAINING

The one word that sticks in my mind about training is *intensity*. Prior to a contest I'm training very fast and very hard. I'm not concerned with handling the heaviest weights, but with pumping the muscles as much as possible, so it's necessary to push a maximum volume of blood through the muscles.

Feeling the muscle and getting your head fully into the area being worked are essential. You have to go through your workout as fast as possible, but still do everything in a productive manner. Rush between sets, but not within a set. In a set, you should do the exercises with continuous tension and peak contraction. Otherwise, it's almost non-stop.

As soon as I put the weight down, I take only a few seconds to get my head into the next movement, and then go again. There's never more than 15-20 seconds rest between sets. Between giant sets, I sometimes take a sip of water, but you can't drink too much, because it may upset your stomach.

I ran one year—in 1977—and got really ripped from it, but too much running can tear down the size of your arms and legs. I don't like to run unless it's absolutely necessary. Still, some bodybuilders I've talked with feel that running is a must before a contest. It depends on your food consumption, so if you're taking in too many calories, you may need to run.

MISCELLANEOUS FACTORS

There are three miscellaneous factors you should take into consideration when ripping up. The first of these is posing practice. By flexing hard and holding the tension in your muscles, you can cut up more than if you didn't. It's almost like taking another workout when you do a half hour or more of posing per day. And by practicing your posing, you can present yourself as a better product than you actually are.

The second miscellaneous factor includes diuretics and laxatives, which some bodybuilders take to flush water out of their bodies a day or two before a show. My opinion of these chemicals is that you have to look healthy on stage, particularly in the line-up. If you look drawn, weak or sickly, I don't think you'll place very high, regardless of how cut you are. If you use diuretics or laxatives, you're bound to end up looking drawn and strung out. If you feel you must resort to a diuretic, I would, but only as a last resort when your timing is off. Otherwise, I prefer not to use them—I'd rather rely on the sun to dehydrate me.

The final miscellaneous factor is mental attitude, and is some ways, this is the most important aspect of your precontest preparations. Peaking is very largely mental. During the middle of the winter once, I was dieting and training very hard, but my mental approach wasn't right to get cut. As a result, I didn't obtain the cuts I should have with the diet I was on.

Close to a contest, however, I begin to visualize how ripped I want to be; and I become ripped, even though the diet is the same or similar to what I was doing during that winter experiment. So, think cuts, if you want cuts.

Getting ripped hasn't been easy for me, but with the four-faceted attack I've just discussed, the process has become less of a burden. Now it has become a semi-exact science. I hope you give some of my methods a try to see if they work for you. See you at the next contest, and you'd best be ripped.

The Reverse Gravity Principle of Training

by Joe Weider

A muscle will achieve its maximum size when it's stimulated with full intensity through the entire range of contraction.

Muscles move bones, and as these bones move through a range of motion, leverages change. The degree of muscular reaction varies according to the changes in leverage.

Muscles help one another. When you lift a weight, some muscles do more work than others due to more advantageous leverage. The muscles that receive the major share of the work will grow the most. Those muscles in a less advantageous position along the line of motion find the weight too heavy to respond with maximum efficiency, and their growth suffers.

Back in the early '50s I wrote about the Reverse Gravity Principle of Training, explaining why reverse resistance could be so effective. The benefit to all the muscles involved in an exercise is not always equally divided, I stated. Reverse resistance can be used to counter this problem.

In order to make a muscle grow, you have to make use of the overload principle. This can be accomplished in more ways than one—e.g., forced reps, supersets.

I learned early that you didn't try to establish detente with muscles. When I was working on Arnold Schwarzenegger's training routines, I had him change his exercises constantly to shock his muscles into responding, to prevent them from adapting. Muscles are very trickly, and soon find the easiest ways of doing various exercises.

So how can you get the entire biceps muscle, for example, to work with maximum intensity through the full range of a curling motion? First of all, you have to use a lot of weight in order to affect the strong middle section of the biceps. But the problem then becomes: how do you get the upper and lower parts of the biceps to handle this excess weight? Simple. By reversing the movement, letting the heavy weight travel slowly downward through the full range of the curling motion.

The upward curl is essentially a ballistic movement. First the weight is boosted off the thighs—however imperceptibly—to gain momentum. In the middle arc of the movement, the biceps exerts its fullest power and continues the momentum upwards. At the top of the arc where the biceps curling power diminishes, the

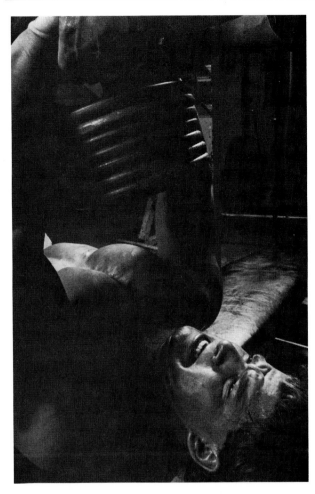

Reverse gravity reps are often done after a training partner helps with forced reps on the positive phase of the movement.

movement is completed, deceptively, by moving the elbows slightly forward, permitting the weight to literally fall the remaining distance to the shoulders. Obviously, only in the middle of arc of the motion does the muscle take in the major load.

If you're capable of getting a 150-pound barbell to the shoulder, you have the start of a heavy curling movement—downward. As the weight descends, you resist, hard, attempting to stall its downward progress. The top, middle and bottom parts of the muscle get a full share of the effort. All the ligaments and tendons get tougher and thicker in a way that doesn't happen when you isolate the parts of the biceps with exercises like Concentration Curls and Incline Curls. You are making the biceps work against 150 pounds in a way not possible with an upward curl of 125 pounds.

There are three ways of using this Reverse Gravity Training Principle:

1. Start at the top of the movement with a heavy weight and lower it slowly all the way down.

2. For the more advanced bodybuilder, a heavy weight can be lowered slowly halfway down, stopped, then raised back to the starting position. Reps can be performed this way, lowering the weight to the bottom position only after completion of the set.

3. A training partner can apply downward pressure on the weight to increase the stress as it's being lowered. This is a kind of "forced reps" in reverse, as you're forced to fight through the slow downward movement.

The trick to this reverse method of training is being able to set up the movements so you can handle them effectively. For example, how would you do reverse Chins Behind The Neck?

Stand on a bench under the chinning bar so that the bar rests across the shoulders. Strap a heavy dumbbell or heavy plate around your waist. Grip the bar at the desired width, lock the lats and raise your feet off the bench. Lower as slowly as you can, resisting hard all the way down to arms' length.

The lats get the full shock of the load right at the beginning of the exercise, in the position of fullest contraction where peak development occurs. When you've lowered yourself to the very bottom, simply stand on the bench and return to the starting position for another rep. You can also leave the feet on the bench during the downward movement, keeping the weight off them as much as possible.

Regular Chins with weights cause you to stall about halfway up after the first few reps (as in Biceps Curls) because you have reached the weak point in the upward movement. Thus, only the muscles exerting power through the lower range of the movement are worked to the limit.

Many top bodybuilders do their Chins without weights in order to get the fullest contraction. Using the Reverse Gravity Training Principle, they could lower themselves with 40%, 50% or even more weight, effectively working the muscles in both the upper and lower ranges of the motion. It's possible for a strong bodybuilder to do reverse-gravity Chins with 150 to 200 pounds strapped around the waist.

After doing the heavy reverse reps, do regular Chins without weight to augment the pump. It's also feasible to do supersets with regular and reverse reps done alternately: one or two reverse reps with a heavy weight, followed by 10 reps of regular Chins, without weight.

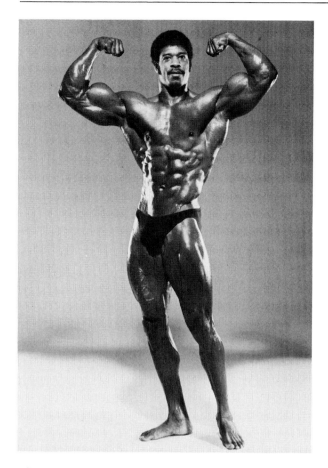

The magnificent biceps of Bill Grant. To get the biceps to work with maximum intensity through the entire range of curling movement, simply reverse the movement.

The Reverse Gravity Principle complements the idea of partial reps (incomplete movements) where the more powerful section of a muscle's range of contraction isn't sacrificed to the weaker sections. For example, you can use much more weight with quarter to half Squats than with full ones.

Also, if you were to do strict Lateral Raises with dumbbells to work the deltoids, you would not be able to budge a heavy enough weight from the side to make the exercise useful. Instead, by raising heavy weights to the horizontal position with a slight throw, and then fighting to lower them slowly, you are in effect doing reverse reps against gravity. The powerful area of contraction at the horizontal level is not sacrificed to the much weaker area a third of the way from the bottom. Thus, you are giving priority to the upper range of motion, permitting the deltoids to handle the heaviest possible weight in this range.

There are a number of reverse gravity exercises that can be done with assistance from a training partner. With the various Lat Pulls, for example, you can overload the pulley and then let the partner give the cable a downward pull. When the handle reaches the finish position near your shoulders or chest, you can slowly return the weight to the starting position.

I suggest you add reverse gravity resistance training to your program. Do about four or five reverse reps for the final set with the heaviest weight possible. The muscles will be thoroughly warmed up from the preceding sets, which will eliminate the possibility of strain. Try a muscle rub to help keep the muscle relaxed and to help remove soreness.

You might keep a chart of the poundages both for the reverse gravity movements and the regular movements. Establish this relationship between them. Don't let one muscle area get ahead of the other. Strive for complete development. Like I said, you can combine reverse movements with regular ones for the same muscle, using the supersets principle.

I developed this reverse gravity idea years ago when I was training with Marvin Eder, Reg Park and Doug Hepburn, all men of super size and strength. It merits a revival. Mike and Ray Mentzer, as well as Casey Viator, have lately been using the principle to increase the intensity of their workouts, and they have all gained greater muscle mass.

Why don't you give this principle a try?

Iso-Tension Concentration for Olympia Muscularity

by Joe Weider

In the rush for super development, it seems that much of the potential for muscle shape and definition is left to chance. The hurry-up-and-get-big idea bypasses some of the more subtle techniques available for quality development.

Many bodybuilders with great physiques fail to reach the top, not from lack of muscle mass, but rather from lack of muscular detail. Whenever a top-seeded contender fails to win, he probably lacked the ultimate in definition, shape and proportion.

That does not mean he was lax in his training. Muscle will do what you want it to do. If you want size, you can get it by using simple exercises and the well-known systems of overload workouts. Getting the ripped-up look that wins contests, however, means you have to coax your muscles beyond the point of maximum pump and tension. A proven method used by today's superstars is the Weider Iso-Tension Concentration Principle.

Some of the old bodybuilding flimflammers like Maxick and Sandow exploited the natural laziness of people and their desire for easy self-improvement by advocating a kind of effortless,

mental concentration method of muscle development. Of course, these men never fully revealed their own fanatical background of training with barbells and dumbbells.

The first of the modern bodybuilders, like Clarence Ross and Ed Theriault, also applied weightless concentration exercises to their weight training programs. These men were in the habit of experimenting, and they found that the weightless contraction of muscle between sets of exercises brought out definition that you couldn't get from weight training alone.

Iso-Tension Concentration is not the same as concentration exercises with weights. Nor is it the same as muscle control, in which the muscles are wiggled or isolated in momentary contraction. Rather, it's a way of building tension in a fully flexed muscle. Iso-Tension Concentration must be used in conjunction with regular weight training. It's not a substitute for weight training. It can be done anytime, anyplace, with or without a mirror.

It's simple to incorporate Iso-Tension Concentration effectively into your regular workout. The muscles, warmed up from the

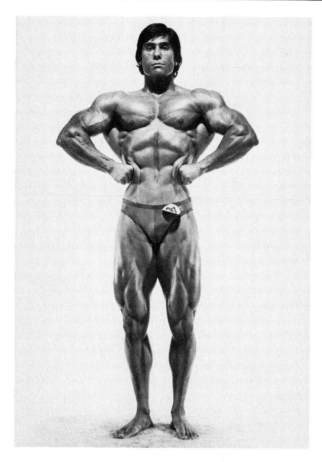

"I heard about Iso-Tension from the Americans and it really works for me," says Jacques Neuville, Mr. Europe.

weight training, will fully respond when you apply iso-tension. You can use this technique to conclude several sets of exercises for a particular body part.

If your regular training schedule calls for four sets of an exercise, complete the four sets. Then, while the muscle is at its peak efficiency and size, continue to flex, contract and crank up the muscle without using weights, forcing the mind and the muscle to fire (i.e., tense) all the fibers in a nearly motionless manner. The tension should be applied intermittently.

The champions have learned to exert this iso-tension in sets of six, holding the tension for three to six seconds, relaxing for a couple of seconds, and tensing again until six reps are completed. They attempt to make each successive stimulus stronger than the previous one. These stimuli act like phantom weights that the brain applies to the muscle when the muscle is fully flexed. The effort can be compared to the forced reps method of training, except that it

involves limited motion and peak contraction.

Many alert champions understand the value of Iso-Tension Concentration exercise. Before a contest, they will do a regular workout in the morning, and in the evening they will do a full-body iso-tension workout for 30 to 60 minutes.

The muscle responds best to iso-tension when it's fully flexed. You can watch this in the mirror. You can literally see the peak of the muscle mount higher as you progress through a series of contractions. The definition and striations begin to show like a photo slowly becoming visible in a developing solution. The entire muscle becomes denser as the peak mounts higher.

It may not happen the first time, but shortly thereafter these concentrated muscle contractions will begin to shape the muscle. They add the finishing touches, details like striations and vascularity, that heavy weights alone cannot provide.

The iso-tension action is explosive. Stimuli are fired into the muscle when it's at peak contraction. The muscle tissue reacts to these sudden, unexpected stimuli by practically climbing out of the skin. It's a marvelous muscle refinement technique for the aspiring bodybuilder!

Remember, however, that you are stressing the muscle beyond the threshold of normal use. To avoid possible cramping or soreness, you must completely extend the muscle or return it to a normal, relaxed position after thoroughly flexing it. You can help alleviate the muscle tension with massage.

Massage helps the blood and lymph flow. It steps up the interchange between the bloodstream and tissue cells. Massage also relieves pain and promotes muscle relaxation by mechanically stretching the muscle. There have even been claims made that massage reduces fat deposits in muscles.

How to get a massage? You can massage yourself, of course. But if you're a top contender for an important title, it would be worthwhile to have a professional masseur work on you once a week, after your heaviest training session.

Franco Columbu has a favorite peak biceps concentration movement. With his elbows forward, he flexes both arms and raises the elbows as high as possible overhead, rotating the wrists inward. The high position is held as long as possible, then relaxed. After that, the tension is repeated for several more reps.

Peak contraction position for the triceps can be achieved by hyperextension of the arm with

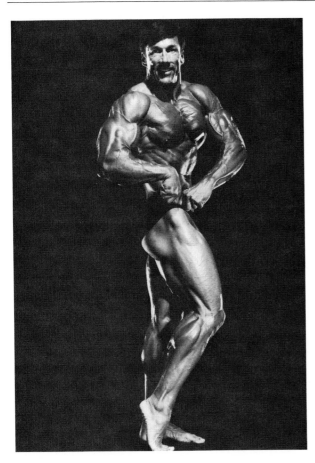

"Joe Weider had me on the Iso-Tension Principle for the last Olympia, and I couldn't believe how much it improved my physique!"
—Boyer Coe, Mr. Universe

the elbow locked straight. A continuing series of peak contractions, breaking the elbow lock slightly each time and returning to the fully locked position with maximum tension, will etch striations and cuts, and will add to triceps density.

The deltoids respond readily to peak contraction. The deltoid is a short, powerful muscle with opposite attachments only inches apart. A lateral raise or handstand will cause the deltoids to lock the shoulder girdle in full peak contraction. By applying iso-tension to a fully flexed delt, alternately tensing and relaxing, you will bring the muscle to its greatest peak. For best results, raise the elbows forward to a horizontal position.

In similar fashion, all the muscles of the body

can be worked with the Iso-Tension Concentration method. Immediately after an abdominal exercise, you can hit the abs with iso-tension by compressing or contracting the muscle. Each block of muscle in the two vertical rows will peak.

For the quadriceps, bring the leg forward in a standing position with the foot slightly to the side. Unlock the knee slightly to make the position comfortable. Maintain balance by leaning the trunk back. Tense the thigh, locking the leg out straight. Hold the tension for six seconds, then relax. Repeat for several reps before lowering the leg.

You can do the above iso-tension exercise following a Squat routine, or you may prefer to do all your weight-free, tension exercises at home when you get back from your workout.

With practice, you will develop optimum positions for the leg biceps, calves, trapezius, rhomboids and other muscles. It's important that you do these Iso-Tension Concentration exercises each training day as a contest approaches.

A lot of bodybuilding contestants don't tense hard enough when they're posing. Iso-Tension Concentration teaches you how to handle your muscles. It gives you better control over them when you're working out. It builds nerve firepower and forces greater muscle peaks. And it enables you to tense all the muscles of the body simultaneously, an important element in contest posing.

Iso-Tension Concentration is not a system that you'll learn overnight. In fact, initial efforts will cause some muscle soreness and stiffness. This technique actually amounts to a new exercise, one which is based on the principle of maximum, sustained contraction. That spells intensity!

Who would have thought that muscle could grow to its present proportions? Muscle has been hit from all angles by the surprise attacks of the relentless Weider muscle-building systems. Discover for yourself how the surprise element of Iso-Tension Concentration can peak your muscles even more and give you that prized definition, shape, contour and control which will put you in full command during a workout or on the posing platform. It's part of the adventure of becoming a super bodybuilder.

Running and the Bodybuilder

by Bill Dobbins

Bodybuilding is a very specialized activity. Strength, endurance, even health, do not matter directly except to the degree that they affect the size, shape and look of the body. The most cardiovascularly conditioned bodybuilder does not win the trophy. As a result, bodybuilders tend to direct all their energy to specific types of training that will be of immediate benefit to them in their quest for greater muscular development, definition and symmetry.

But overall conditioning may prove to be more important in bodybuilding than previously thought. Specificity of training is as important in bodybuilding as it is in any other sport, but there is also some evidence that the health of the body as a whole—including heart, lungs and circulatory system—may have a decisive effect on the development of muscular hypertrophy over an extended period of time.

Really hard training drains the body of energy. After years of this kind of abuse, the body may no longer be able to replace this lost energy in sufficient quantities to allow hard training to continue. This is one of the causes of "burning out." It has both a physical and psychological component. When your energy levels ebb, you feel depressed and unmotivated. The results are poor workouts and a lack of progress in physical development.

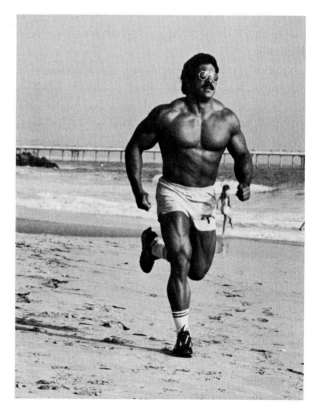

Ray Mentzer (shown here on a Southern California beach) and his brother, Mike, both include running in their training—as an aid to cutting up and keeping their weight down.

It may take years for these symptoms to manifest themselves. However, bodybuilding careers are becoming longer and longer as new opportunities for competition open up, especially those involving prize money for professionals. Therefore, it makes sense for bodybuilders to begin some kind of program for "preventive maintenance" before they start to experience any difficulties.

Part of this program would involve proper diet and such things as avoiding extended low-carbohydrate diets or anything else detrimental to the system. Another would be to develop a safe and sane attitude toward drugs. Anabolic steroids taken in large doses over extended periods of time (especially when no physician is supervising the program) cannot help but have an injurious effect on the body. Also, there is the need to keep the cardio-respiratory system in good shape. One of the best ways to do this is by running.

Many bodybuilders are wary of including running in their training programs. For one thing, they are afraid of losing muscular size, but when running is done in moderate amounts, this is not a real problem. According to J. A. Feliciano, long, endurance-type running has an effect on the quality of muscle.

If you look at a long distance runner's legs, you can see that the muscles are long and slender. This type of running actually changes the physiology of the muscle. It's obvious that these changes are not desirable for bodybuilders." Instead of LSD (long slow distance), Feliciano recommends running shorter distances at faster speeds. "A mile is a good distance, if you keep up the pace. Better still, try running in sand, up a hill, or running up steps. All of this has to be done intensely to deliver the trauma to the legs that will build them up."

Hard bursts of speed and effort have the double advantage of helping to build muscularity in the legs while improving cardiovascular conditioning at the same time. The endurance this provides has only indirect effect on the endurance qualities of the upper body, but it does improve the ability of the heart and lungs to deliver oxygen to the entire system. This will improve the upper body's capacity to develop endurance through hard training, and good endurance allows for more training intensity.

Many top bodybuilders currently include some type of running in their training schedules. Robby Robinson, for example, runs a mile or so in Palisades Park, a block from Gold's Gym,

before starting his workout. "Running makes me feel good," Robby explains. "It gets my heart pumping, blood flowing through my body, and I feel really ready to put a lot of energy into training." Robby also points out that running has another advantage: It burns up calories and produces a lot of water loss, both conducive to helping the bodybuilder cut up.

"I'm all for it," says Bill Pearl, whose longevity as a top bodybuilder attests to the fact that whatever he has been doing works. "Running helps in weight loss and lets you get cut up that much faster. I think it really helps my muscularity. A lot of bodybuilders I have trained and worked with have been runners: Chris Dickerson, for example, Jim Morris and Dennis Tinerino." Pearl trains very early in the morning and usually runs afterward. However, he does not think that is the ideal system.

"I was involved in a project that determined it is better to run first, before your workout, than to wait and do your running afterward. My own schedule makes that difficult for me, but I would recommend running before the workout to anyone who has the opportunity." Like other bodybuilders, Bill Pearl is careful not to run on the same day he has a leg workout planned.

Mike Mentzer is another top competitor who believes in running. "I go a couple of miles two or three times a week," he says. "Primarily I use it to keep my weight down. With my short, intense workouts I don't burn as many calories in the gym as some other bodybuilders. So running is good for helping me cut up, as well as keeping my heart and lungs in good condition."

Anybody interested in learning proper running techniques has a multitude of sources to learn from these days. There are close to a dozen popular books on the subject as well as magazines available on newsstands. However, for those who are not interested in buying a book or magazine on running, here are a few important pointers.

—WEAR RUNNING SHOES. Running shoes are different from tennis shoes. Tennis shoes give more side-to-side support, while running shoes are designed to cushion the feet and legs from the jarring of running.

—START OUT SLOWLY. It takes a while to build up endurance. But for most bodybuilders, who are in pretty good shape in the first place, building up the "wind" does not take very long. The problem is that very soon the lungs outlast the legs. That is, they can keep going so long that they can deliver more trauma to the legs than the legs can stand. This results in soreness or worse. If you have to lay off two or three weeks because of injury you will have to start all over again, so better build up gradually and give the legs a chance to get used to that kind of stress.

—*PICK YOUR SURFACE.* Concrete is harder on the legs than is grass. The harder the surface on which you run, the more chance of injury. Run on a soft surface if you can. If you cannot, then limit your running until your legs, ankles and feet get used to the shock.

—*PROTECT YOUR LUNGS.* When you run, a lot of air goes through your lungs, so you should be careful it is as clean as possible. On days when there is a lot of pollution, run early in the morning or late in the evening. Avoid running alongside highways where you are constantly breathing car exhaust.

—*RUN BY TIME, NOT DISTANCE.* Most people cannot estimate distances like one or two miles with any degree of accuracy. So instead of running pre-set distances, try running by your watch. Pick a good pace, then run for 15 minutes without a break. Next time, try for 20. It should take between 20 and 30 minutes to run three miles. After you can run for 30 minutes without stopping, don't run longer; just try running a little faster for the same length of time.

—*NOTICE THE PAIN.* There are different kinds of pain. One kind comes from a buildup of lactic acid in the muscles. This produces the same kind of "burn" you get doing high reps in the gym. The other kind of pain comes from injury to joints, muscles, ligaments and sometimes bone. Do not try to run through this latter kind of pain. It will only get worse. Instead, suspend your running workouts for a while and rest the painful area.

—*STRETCH AND WARM UP.* When you run you subject your leg muscles to fast, hard effort. If they are not in condition, this can lead to injury. To avoid this, do some stretching exercises before you run. And then start out slow until the blood gets flowing freely to your lower extremities. Incidentally, most running coaches advise some stretching afterwards as well.

Running burns up a minimum of 100 calories a mile. Therefore, a half hour of running should burn up at least 300 calories. This may not seem like very much. At this rate, it would take 11 or 12 days of running to burn up a pound of fat. However, when a bodybuilder is dieting seriously, every pound counts. After lowering your caloric intake as far as you can, it becomes impossible to lose any weight by cutting back any further. Therefore, the running can be decisive. Additionally, it leads to water loss, and running is also helpful in suppressing the appetite.

Kal Szkalak believes running has another advantage. "Just before a contest, when you are on a diet and the nervous energy is building up, running is a good way of channeling that energy into constructive directions." Kal runs three times a week anyway, but he has noticed that running helps him to avoid any of the problems a bodybuilder can experience while preparing for a contest. Unused energy has a way of developing into anxiety unless it is expended. Since a positive attitude is so important both in training and in contest presentation, running can serve a valuable function for the competitive bodybuilder.

Not all bodybuilders believe in running. Pete Grymkowski, for example, thinks that running is detrimental to bodybuilding. "When you run you are constantly jarring your body," he says, "and what this does is increase the pull of gravity on the body. This exerts a lot of force on the muscles, tearing at the supporting structures, and tends to make them sag."

But the consensus seems to be that running done in moderation is good for the bodybuilder. The only problem is that the athlete only has so much energy to go around. If too much is expended in running (or swimming, riding a bike and anything else), it will interfere with training. Experiment by running at different times, different days, and different numbers of times a week to find out what suits you. Remember, you may use more energy preparing for a competition than you do the rest of the year, so you may have to be ready to vary your running schedule.

All other things being equal (which they never are), the better conditioned, healthier athlete is going to be the better bodybuilder and will be able to maintain his physique for a longer time. Running is one good way to make that happen for you.

My Way

by Ed Corney
The Master Poser

Posing is an extension of self.

You can spend thousands of hours sweating in a gym and eat only water-packed tuna for weeks. You can end up looking like a work of art. You can do all this and still fall flat on your face at a contest.

Only by extending your personality through effective and dramatic posing can you let the judges and audience identify with you and know exactly what you've gone through to reach the top. Add great posing to years in the gym and months on a tight diet, and you are sure to carry home some new trophies.

I vividly recall my first competition and the trepidations I experienced at the thought of getting up on stage to pose. My training partner and I had been working out at Bob's Gym in Fremont, California. I was 32 and hadn't really considered competing in anything, but then the gym decided to promote the first Mr. Fremont contest for its members.

My partner and I trained like dogs, threw together a few poses and stood backstage ready to go on. I was so shaky that I had to take a couple of belts of vodka to generate the nerve to get up there. After hitting a few hasty shots, I jumped off stage, relieved that the ordeal was

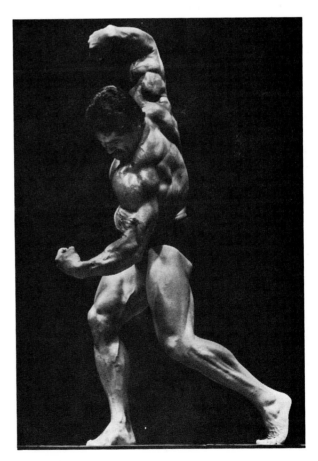

Ed Corney
The Master Poser

41

over. You can imagine my surprise and elation when I was awarded first place and my partner took second!

Today I laugh at how inept I was in that first contest. Today I *live* to get up on stage and communicate with my audience. No sensation in my life can equal that of being at the Olympia in top shape and flowing powerfully, yet gracefully, through my routine. I live to hear 4000 throats screaming for more!

In the 13–14 years I've been competing, my posing has undergone numerous changes. After that first Mr. Fremont competition, I was ashamed at how quickly I'd gotten on and off stage. Here I was, a contest winner who looked like he was afraid to compete! Deep down I wanted to savor the moments up on stage, so it was necessary to extend my routine over a longer period of time. This was accomplished the same way everyone does it—by adding more poses.

Soon I was winning all the shows in Northern California. At that time the only important factor to me was hitting each pose to show myself at my best. Unfortunately, hundreds of bodybuilders are still stuck at this rudimentary level of posing development. They completely ignore the showmanship and transitions between poses, so their routine looks very static and their movements between poses are often fidgety and clumsy.

I was after something more, and while spending at least an hour per day on posing, I hit upon a few transitions that excited me. My philosophy at the time was that when you were up on stage, the posing was as important as the training, so why not spend as much time on posing as in the gym? The hundreds of nights I spent in front of the mirror gave birth to the smooth transitions between poses.

Roughly a third of my time on stage is spent moving between poses. These movements are fully choreographed, the same as a dance production on television. Indeed, posing is very much like dancing. I've taken several series of ballet classes to improve my stage presentation. It's easy to relate the balance requirements and arm movements of ballet to a heroic style of contest posing. The flowing nature of ballet is very similar to posing.

When posing, every part of my body is crucial to the overall picture, and every expression, every gesture is precisely choreographed. Have you ever thought about the expression on your face as you pose? Your facial expression can convey joy, triumph, power and a full command of the situation. Or your face can reflect boredom, fright and lack of self-assurance. Which expressions do you think would most turn on a judge or someone in the audience?

Foot position is vital to balance. Without a solid foot stance, you can stumble all over the stage, and without placing your feet precisely, you'll have difficulty maintaining your balance when pivoting. If you've seen me pose and like the pivoting double biceps and archer poses toward the end of my routine, you can appreciate the fact that having my feet only a half inch off the correct marks will destroy the power and grace of these movements. Just a half inch off and I look like an oaf!

Hand position is equally crucial. An open hand, for example, conveys a feeling of grace, while a closed fist has always been symbolic of power. I even enclose my thumb in my fist for greater emphasis of this power.

Melding grace with power gives me a balanced routine. I do this by opening my hands as I move and then clenching them in the actual poses.

Some of my arm gestures are intended to symbolically pull the audience into my routine. I don't actually wave someone toward me with a big gesture of my arm, but there are several arm movements that can be interpreted as "gathering" gestures. The audience is subconsciously gathered up and pulled toward me. Then it can better share my euphoria as I pose.

There are many other facets of posing that I explore in my posing course. Since space is limited, I'd suggest that you order my posing course, or perhaps attend one of my posing seminars.

In the meantime, there are several suggestions I can make to improve your posing. To begin with, I consistently spend as much time practicing my posing as I do actually training. This means I'm posing up to three hours per day before the Olympia. The posing improves from all this, of course, and my muscle hardness also gets better from the constant tension.

I've arranged three large mirrors in a manner that allows me to see every pose from all angles. This can be invaluable, particularly in learning the "feel" of a straight back shot. It may feel right and look like *guano*, or it may look best only when it feels totally off. These things can only be determined if you can see yourself in the same way the judges see you.

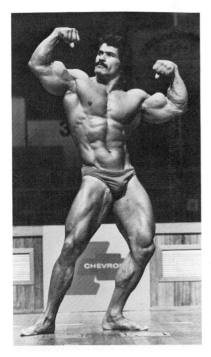

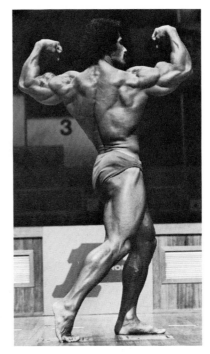

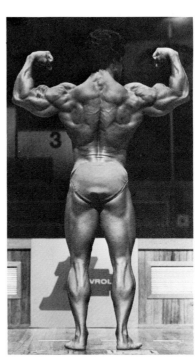

"It's been said that I look good from every angle. If that's true, it's because I train for good proportions, and chose poses that suit my individual body."

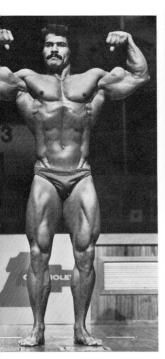

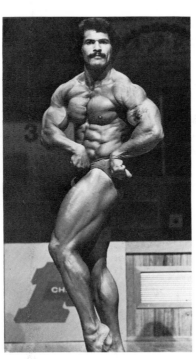

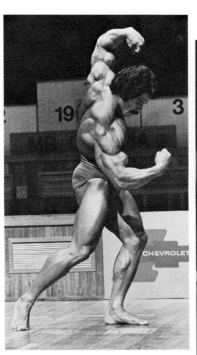

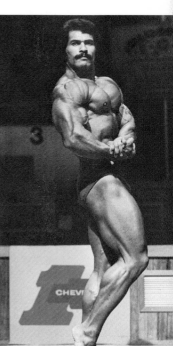

"My transitions are half of the presentation, and the poses are momentarily static interludes in a dancelike routine. Showmanship is often over looked by even Olympian posers."

I also set up a posing lamp and have a tape deck handy. The light has to be similar to that at a contest, or you may be showing something you don't want to on stage. The music helps my posing rhythm. Usually I pose on stage to Frank Sinatra's "My Way," with which I can identify thoroughly, but at home I use a variety of music.

All of the posing I do is coordinated with what I see in the numerous photos taken of me at contests and exhibitions. You should be very critical of what you see in your own photos. *Never* overlook a weak body part. Bring it up, and look for poses that can hide it until it is up. Ultimately, however, you will need good proportions, or you'll never make it to the top.

If you practice hard and long, you won't fall on your face at your next contest. You'll be able to say, "I posed and posed well. I did it my way!"

Cold Cure for Muscle Injury

by Dr. Franco Columbu

Ice has been shown to be superior to heat as a simple, safe and effective therapy after soft-tissue injury. It can cut weeks off the recovery time by reducing swelling and increasing deep circulation in the area of the injury.

Heat, on the other hand, increases the swelling. While heat also increases the circulation, it does so only in the surface area of an injury. Increased deep circulation, coupled with exercise, is the best way to clear out the debris of injury.

The effectiveness of ice should come as good news to bodybuilders, who hate the long rehabilitation process following a muscle injury. Muscle strains are a well-known condition of life in weight training and the treatment of such soft-tissue injuries should be considered part of the recuperative process.

Ice therapy, which is known as cryotherapy, or sometimes cryokinetics, is often confused with ice first-aid treatment. There are important differences.

Ice packs, as a first-aid treatment, are left in place up to an hour at a time during the first 24 to 48 hours following an injury. This is reasonably effective in controlling blood clots and continued injury to the tissue from lack of circulation and oxygen.

Cryotherapy rehabilitation, as different from first-aid, begins on the first or second day of the injury—depending on the severity of the injury. The technique is relatively simple, and all variations lead to the same conclusions. After six to 12 minutes of chilling through ice massage, ice towels or iced whirlpools, the athlete takes advantage of the partial anesthesia offered by the chilling to put himself through active range-of-motion exercises until pain returns. When the pain comes back, the cycle of ice application followed by exercise is repeated.

As mentioned earlier, ice therapy can save days or weeks of rehabilitation time. Research has shown that responses to ice massage are all of considerable benefit to the injured athlete. The most important responses are initial vasoconstriction, later deep-tissue vasodilation, reduction in muscle spasm, and limited thermal anesthesia.

Here is what happens during each of these responses:

1. *Vasoconstriction*—During the first nine to 16 minutes of ice therapy, the affected area undergoes a reduction in blood flow through both reflexive vasoconstriction and blood viscosity. In other words, the blood gets thicker as the blood vessels get narrower. Local swelling is reduced and less inflammation appears.

2. *Vasodilation*—As the ice therapy continues, a sudden deep-tissue dilation of the blood vessels occurs, lasting four to six minutes. This greatly raises the local temperature as a defense against the prolonged cold. The blood vessels then reconstrict again. This, in turn, is followed by blood vessel dilation in a 15- to 30-minute cycle.

3. *Muscle Spasm*—Muscle cramping is reduced. Deep tendon reflexes also diminish, and the muscle becomes more relaxed.

4. Limited Anesthesia—Five to 10 minutes of ice packs will reduce pain in a pulled or strained muscle/ligament to a level that permits active exercise through an increased range of motion. Ice numbs the pain. When ice is applied, the athlete first feels intense cold, burning and aching. Then the thermal anesthesia takes effect. The pain-killing effect of ice lasts much longer than the effects of heat treatment.

EXERCISE IS IMPORTANT

The speed of recovery of a muscle or ligament injury is determined by the amount of the swelling and the speed with which the body mobilizes the debris. Ice limits the initial damage, and ice and exercise help move the debris out.

The injury must be exercised to increase the circulation. The reasoning is simple though: the greater the blood flow to an area, the greater the removal of waste products. This has always been the purpose of the Weider Maximum Muscle Pump Principle in bodybuilding training.

The rehabilitative exercise should be voluntary and active. Use the maximum resistance that can be handled without pain. If the movement hurts, it should be avoided. Rotary movements of joints and muscle groups should be emphasized. The injured area should be relaxed before attempting exercise.

Ice therapy can work so quickly that athletes who might otherwise be lost for an entire season can sometimes be back in action within one or two weeks. A leading investigator in ice therapy, Robert J. Moore, Ph.D, head athletic trainer and professor of physical education at San Diego

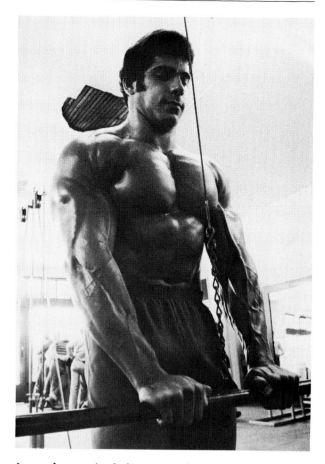

Ice and excercise help more debris out.

State University, offers the following techniques:

1. *Ice Massage*—The injured area is massaged with ice (in the form of an ice ball or cube) for five to 10 minutes. The massaging action should be gentle.

2. *Ice Bath*—The injured part is immersed in a container of flaked ice and water for about five to six minutes. The temperature should be approximately 40°F. This technique can be used mainly for injuries of the distal joints, such as knees, ankles, elbows and hands.

3. *Ice Towel*—The towels are immersed in 40°F. ice water, wrung out, and placed on the entire injured area. The technique is best suited for use with exercise—the athlete can be exercising while receiving treatment. This is a good treatment technique for areas such as the back, chest and thighs.

4. *Ice Pack*—The injured area is covered with a pack, which is made by putting a layer of crushed ice between two terry cloth towels. The ice pack should remain on for 15-20 minutes. This technique is especially useful in cases of severe injury where pain and/or edema are

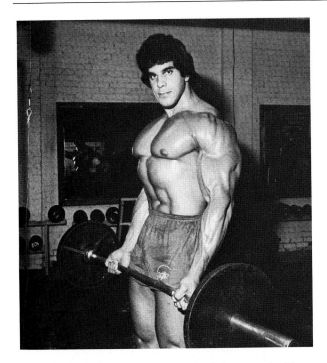

If a bodybuilder injured his biceps doing a curl with 100 pounds, he would use less weight for curl movements.

significant problems. Therapeutic exercises are started after the ice pack is removed, or they can be done while the pack is in place.

An injured athlete should never be returned to intense physical activity while under the anesthetic effect of ice therapy. If a bodybuilder injured his biceps doing a curl with 100 pounds, he would use less weight for curl movements while the biceps was undergoing cold treatment.

When an acutely injured ligament or tendon is chilled, the physical characteristics of its collagen are altered. It becomes less stretchable and tends to contract. This condition benefits the injury during elevation and compression, but it may cause more serious injury if stress is continued.

Dr. Moore says, "Cryotherapy is probably the safest of treatments, but there must be a thorough evaluation of the injury, including X-ray if there is any question, followed by 24 to 48 hours of ice, compression and elevation before the active range-of-motion exercises begin."

Ice therapy is easy and economical. A cylindrical ice cake frozen in a Styrofoam cup can be held in the hand, and the injured area massaged directly with the ice. A bucket of ice water or a towel pack with shaved ice are also simple applications. Frozen gel packs are almost as good as ice.

The athlete can treat himself until he can do exercises without pain. Such self-treatment can be a psychological stimulant to recovery. And the simplicity of the treatment defies mistakes.

The following case is cited by Dr. Moore:

A football player suffered a complete dislocation of the elbow. The dislocation was reset and the involved arm was placed in a sling.

The injury normally would have required five weeks in the sling, and the player would be lost for the season. Two days after injury, however, ice therapy (immersion) was begun under the direction of the team physician, and rehabilitative exercises performed. Full, pain-free motion was achieved on the fourth day! On the fifth day, the athlete was able to perform two Chin-Ups and five Push-Ups without pain. Nine days after the injury, the attending physician allowed the player to resume full participation in football.

The athlete remained on the rehabilitation program for the rest of the season, but was able to play as a regular team member without re-injury.

The above are heartening facts and statistics to the hard-training bodybuilder who sustains a muscle injury, especially if it happens in the shadow of an approaching contest. He can treat himself, and the treatment is cheap and simple. Conceivably, he could well be into full-bore training after several days, rather than weeks or even months of delay.

Ice therapy should rate high on the list of recuperative processes for bodybuilders. It seems to reduce injuries from being tragedies to being mere nuisances.

Machines:
Scientific Shortcut to Success?

by Bill Dobbins

"You realize, Sean," I said, "that a lot of bodybuilders would agree with these criticisms." He smiled, nodded and continued to read the article that had been sent to Joe Weider attacking the efficacy of training with machines in general and Nautilus equipment in particular.

Sean Harrington owns and operates the Nautilus Fitness and Training Center in Brentwood, a suburb of Los Angeles. I interviewed him at the request of Joe Weider, who wanted to make sure *Muscle & Fitness* readers heard both sides of this controversial question.

"I know it," Sean replied. "Bodybuilders are traditionalists. If something has worked in the past, they're reluctant to try anything new. I'll admit, that makes a certain amount of sense."

But it doesn't mean he agrees. Sean and the other Nautilus believers are convinced that their equipment provides the fastest and most efficient way of developing both enhanced strength and muscular hypertrophy. They can point to a large body of research which tends to support their position. Unfortunately, what they can't produce is a single champion bodybuilder whose physique was created totally on Nautilus

equipment. That, they say, is because the machines are still new, and bodybuilders don't as yet have enough confidence in them to train with the Nautilus machines exclusively. But to Sean Harrington and Nautilus creator Arthur Jones, it is just a matter of time.

"First of all," Sean said, "dealing with the question of whether exercise movements take place in only one plane. In fact the normal path, the normal way your body works is in circles. No body part works in a straight line. The joint is a ball and socket, and the range of motion depends on that particular socket. Our equipment follows the natural line of the body in that it does work in a circular path." With free weights you have to work in more or less a straight line to keep the weight in balance, and this, Sean says, is a less natural way to move.

"In an exercise like a bicep curl," he said, "you can't do it strictly with a free weight. When you get working heavy, you'll find you tend to lift the weight in a straight line, too. On Nautilus curl machines that doesn't happen."

Sean emphasizes that the purpose of Nautilus equipment is to isolate and strengthen the individual muscles of the body. He admits that

48

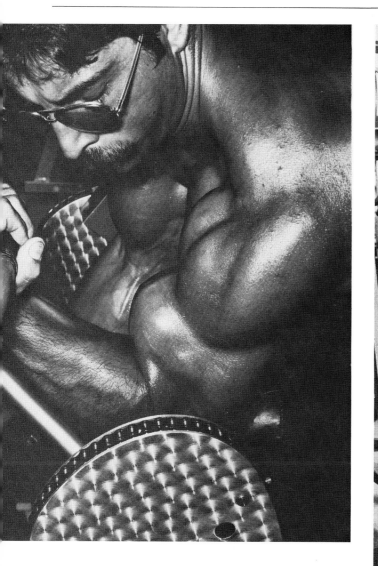

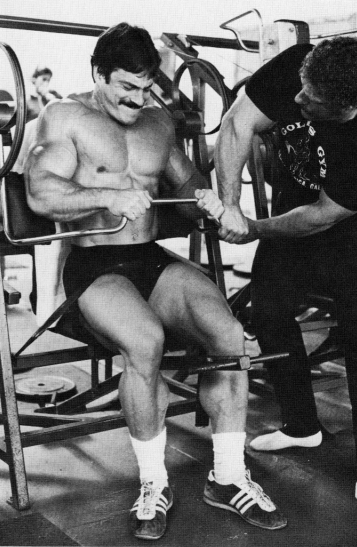

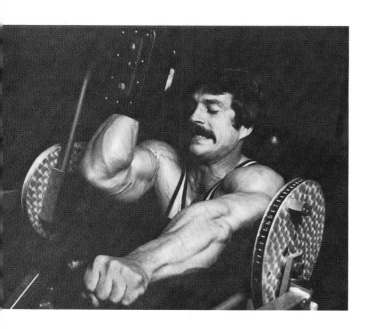

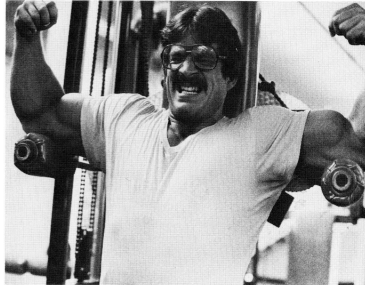

working on his machines won't develop skill and coordination. To develop skill, he says, you have to work on that particular skill.

"If a person was going to become a powerlifter or an Olympic lifter, the best way for him to become that would be to lift weights. It wouldn't be to work on Nautilus equipment. Part of his routine could be working with Nautilus, but it's like a football player. He can use Nautilus equipment to condition him for football, but if he never practices football, he'll never be any good at it." Sean points out that people who train on Nautilus machines and then, when they go back to working with free weights find themselves weaker, are forgetting about the skill factor.

"There's a tremendous amount of technique involved in weight lifting. It's obvious as soon as you step into a gym. The strongest person is not necessarily the best powerlifter. We can help a powerlifter get stronger, but we can't help his technique."

For example, Sean points out, an exercise like the bench press involves a lot of timing and balance, but it is not necessarily a good representation of pure strength. This becomes more evident in Olympic events such as the clean and jerk. Nautilus provides a better indication of the absolute strength of any given muscle, according to Sean.

"Bodybuilders get very frustrated when they come into the center," Sean says. "They're used to lifting weights and, whenever you do, you're bound to cheat some. Since you can't cheat very easily using Nautilus, you're not going to be able to use as much weight. That's very ego-deflating and it bothers a lot of bodybuilders. I can see why, too. I don't blame them. But we're not trying to help people lift weights, we're trying to help their bodies and their sports performance. Bodybuilders would be a lot better off if they remembered they weren't weightlifters and concentrated purely on developing their muscles."

Another advantage of Nautilus exercise, says Sean, is that it involves a full range of motion that not only increases the overall strength of a muscle throughout its entire length, but also develops greater flexibility. If you're concerned about enhancing general athletic skill, as well as preventing injury, Sean feels that increased flexibility is absolutely essential. This, he believes, answers any questions about Nautilus training not really helping athletic ability.

I reminded Sean at this point that some of the criticism that *Muscle & Fitness* would be publishing involved the principle of variable resistance, practically the foundation of the Nautilus design: Do the machines really reflect the varying strength curve of each muscular movement?

"I feel that the worst person in the world to talk about strength curves with would be a bodybuilder, because he's completely changed his natural strength curve. Years of lifting with short range-of-motion exercises, using muscles that would normally not be brought into play, have altered his strength curve radically. And that means that a bodybuilder or weightlifter's power curve may not agree with the Nautilus machine's cam, which is designed to reflect the muscle's *natural* capability. There was a lot of testing done to determine what that natural strength curve is."

Sean believes that most people don't understand just how sophisticated a Nautilus device is. They think it produces variable resistance along a constant curve, making the weight heavier at the bottom, lighter at the top. This, he says, is not always the case.

"It changes with each machine," explained Sean. "Some cams produce more resistance somewhere near the middle and less at the end. Each of the cams is different. They all work different strength curves. And the cam isn't the only thing that varies the resistance. Don't forget, there's also a counterweight. At the end of a movement where it might seem the cam is producing greater resistance, in fact there may be less weight because the counterweight has come into play. It completely changes that resistance."

In spite of all this evidence to support the idea of Nautilus training, Sean is convinced that few bodybuilders will actually convert to an all-Nautilus training routine. The reason, he believes, is that bodybuilders get addicted to the training itself, completely apart from the results. They learn to like spending the hours in the gym and the feeling of doing many repetitions with the weights. Nautilus training involves workouts of 20 minutes, three times a week. It does not satisfy a "trainaholic."

"Bodybuilders don't want to believe that they are actually limiting their progress by so much training," said Harrington. "It's true of a lot of athletes as well. The point is, when you get strong enough, you can put so much stress on your body that it takes several days to recover. Your recovery time doesn't get much shorter as you get in condition, so the more advanced you get, the *less* you have to train. Even though bodybuilders get results here, they miss the longer routine at the bodybuilding gym. It just comes down to whether or not you consider results the most important thing."

"What about the possibility of training injuries? You hear a lot of criticism leveled at the machines—that they cause arthritic conditions, that they put an undo amount of strain on tendons and ligaments, and so forth."

Not true, he says. In fact, Nautilus equipment is often used for physical rehabilitation, because it allows you to isolate and work certain muscles to the exclusion of others. None of the members of his fitness center (who train under the supervision of Sean and his staff) has ever developed problems of this kind, he states emphatically. Arthritic conditions in particular, he said, benefit from Nautilus training due to the full-range of motion involved and the additional flexibility created.

"A bodybuilder, however," Sean is careful to note, "may find that he is hurting himself at one particular point of the range of motion. This may be because he's never worked the full range of motion before and he's overdeveloped a certain part of that range.

"He's developed very great strength in that middle portion which is out of proportion with the rest—he can't handle the weight when the machine forces him to use the part he's not used to. So, in order to do it right, he'd have to start his program by using a lighter weight until he develops range proportionally. And what bodybuilder is going to want to do that?"

At Joe Weider's request, I checked with an expert in sports medicine to see if the medical community agreed with Sean Harrington's assessment of the safety record compiled by the Nautilus machinery. Dr. Walter Jekot treats a great number of bodybuilders and weightlifters at his Hollywood office, and he is deeply involved in the developing field of sports medicine. I asked him about Nautilus-related injuries.

"I've never had a single case," he admitted, "that to my knowledge was an injury incurred while training with Nautilus equipment. Also, I don't recall any articles in the various sports medicine journals that relate cases involving such

injuries. However, let me point out that this kind of equipment is relatively new and it hasn't been around long enough for us to make any really good assessments of its potential to cause injuries. All we can do is to keep an eye on developments and watch for any problems that might arise in the future."

Dr. Jekot does believe, however, that in any system depending on maximum intensity for an exercise—whether it's training for powerlifting with free weights or a Nautilus program—the closer you work toward your limit, the more liable you are to become injured. "I see a lot of pulled muscles, shoulder separations, elbow and knee problems. Some are obviously more serious than others, but whenever you put any type of strain on the body, you take a certain risk. I don't say that to deter anyone from athletics, but there is always some risk of injury involved."

After my session with Sean, I thought about the things he'd told me. I don't know enough to say for certain whether he is correct in whole or in part, or whether the criticisms that Nautilus is often subjected to will be proven or discarded. Overall, I thought he made a lot of sense, but it's going to take a lot more research—by people other than Nautilus researchers in Florida—to make a final determination.

It is true that bodybuilding has developed on a hit-or-miss basis throughout its relatively short history. We frequently do things because that's the way they've always been done, or because that's the sort of program someone we admire has followed. True, some amazing physiques have been developed. The question is, could they have been developed just as far or in a shorter period of time using some other kind of training method?

In this day and age of scientific progress, the answer is yes, but I don't know what those training methods might be. The principles behind Arthur Jones' Nautilus machines might be a great step forward—then again, maybe not.

Someday—sooner or later—we will discover still better ways to train. And you can bet that most of us will reject them because they don't "feel" right, even though feeling is a poor way to assess what is going on in such a complex biochemical mechanism as the human body.

Until science lets us know conclusively, it's the best we can do.

Machines:
A Pitfall on the Way to Progress?

by George Elder
Strength Coach
University of New Hampshire

THE MACHINE AGE

As of late, the "machine age" has threatened to dominate the field of progressive resistance exercise programs. All around us, we hear of great achievements realized through the use of the many weight training machines now on the market. Most companies promise a maximal result in gain within a minimal amount of time. It has been my experience that almost every athlete, in any sport, seeks some great method to achieve superiority over his opponent. All the above companies promise to meet that need expediently. It's easy to see how attractive these machines become when we consider the above.

Most of these companies offer a plethora of studies and data to back their claims. Many of these reports glow with tremendous results that are to be obtained by use of their products. These studies are written in a professional and convincing manner and can be quite persuasive.

Add to this word of mouth and testimonials (so prevalent now-a-days), and one can easily see why these companies have been so successful. These companies are dealing with a market whose constituents are eager and easily sold. This is in no way to say that the market is ignorant, it is merely expedient.

I have been involved in all forms of weight training for at least 10 years. During this time, my understanding of words such as *size* and *strength* have achieved new meanings. When a 198-pounder cleans and jerks 425 pounds or a 350-pounder squats with 920 pounds, that's size and strength.

From my experience, *no* machine or group of machines put out by *any* company comes close to the results with regards to strength and size that can be achieved from free-weights. Few, if any machines, offer the capacity to train an athlete athletically.

One might ask how I could possibly state the above, in light of recent studies. My answer is, very easily. I don't believe all that I read and very little of what I hear. To back up my opinion, I offer only my personal observations.

Four summers ago, I trained extensively on "N" machines. My workouts were performed exactly as prescribed on the literature. Over the course of three months, I became quite proficient at handling substantial amounts of plates on these machines. While my weight didn't increase, I noticed that my definition did. At the end of three months I was able to handle all the plates on certain machines for up to 17 repetitions. Of course I thought my strength had improved dramatically.

Upon returning to school, I experienced a rude awakening. My pre-summer free weight workout was all I could do, because I lacked access to any machines. Upon trying to perform the same workouts after two weeks of free weight pre-conditioning, I found myself completely incapable of handling the weights or reps I had done three months before. This applied to *all* my movements. As an example of a before and after, consider the following:

Before: Standing Olympic Press: 350 pounds maximum

Workout #1: 185 X 5, 245 X 3, 285 X 3, 315 X 3, 225 X 8

After: Standing Olympic Press: 305 pounds maximum

Workout #1: 185 X 5, 225 X 3, 265 X 3, 305 X miss, 305 X 1, 225 X 6.

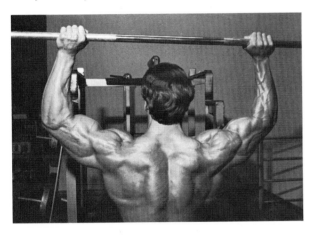

It took me two months to get back to form. In essence, I wasted three months training time, plus two months reconditioning myself.

Five months down the drain gave me a bad taste for machines. I figured that maybe my results were unusual and just a fluke. Maybe the machines were good, but for some reason they didn't work for me. So I decided to run a mini-test.

Over the next summer, June through August, six subjects trained exclusively on the "N" machines. I took special care to test them on free weights very carefully before they left and when they came back. Due to time limitations, I could only retest the bench press but the results of this mini-test were quite conclusive. Five of the six did worse upon retesting and one did the same. The average loss in the bench was 24.5 pounds. One individual lost 55 pounds in his bench. The average body weight gain was 2.58 pounds with markedly improved hypertrophy. These athletes looked stronger but they were

weaker. It took between six and nine weeks to get their strength levels up to pre-summer standards.

It was interesting to note that all of the athletes complained about a lack of ability to balance the bar. All displayed uneven extention and very poor lock out. In effect, they had lost much of their capacity to handle a freely moving object in a coordinated and effective fashion.

Since most objects encountered in athletics are freely moving (i.e. opposing players), I became quite concerned with the athlete's performances. Whenever we deal with most machines, we are talking about dealing in fixed planes. Usually there is an axis of movement which can only take place in one plane, and this limits a machine's capacity to fully develop the muscle. Most machines are worked on a very slow movement basis, so the athlete doesn't have to worry about balance, coordination, speed or timing when he trains. But since these are all the attributes we expect from an athlete, why shouldn't he train to achieve strength and size gains in an athletic fashion? Machines, by nature, do not allow an athlete to work in a truly athletic fashion.

On the other hand, there are the much maligned free weights. These devices have to be lifted with some degree of athletic ability due to their multi-planar nature. When one performs a clean, he uses a great many muscles in an organized and athletic way. Such exercises have a proven capacity to improve strength in an *athletic* manner.

Free weights better prepare the athlete to handle freely moving objects—the kind he will deal with in his given sport. They are instrumental in the development of balance, coordination, speed and timing.

Our view of athletics should include a "total" picture. Strength, speed, size and many other factors go into making an athlete. When training an athlete for a specific purpose, i.e. strength, one must keep this total picture in mind. We cannot isolate a certain muscle and train it in a very specific manner. We must train a group of muscles and develop them in an athletic manner.

THE VALUE OF VARIABLE RESISTANCE

One of the biggest selling points used by many companies who produce weight training machines is the purported advantage of variable resistance. These companies claim that their devices have the capability to automatically increase the amount of resistance in the final ranges of a given movement. The main reason given is that it is necessary to increase the resistance in the final stages of a movement due to the increased skeletal leverage a subject has at that point of the exercise. These companies point out that this makes their products superior to free weights, because free weights are not capable of working a muscle equally throughout its full range.

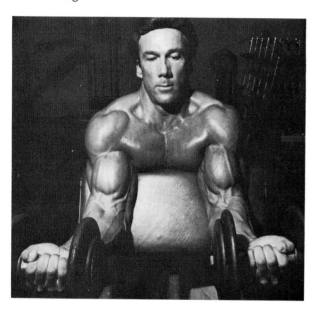

At face value this seems to make sense. In the squat, there is little work for the muscle to do in the final third of the lift. But many exercises are *not* the strongest towards the end of a given movement. In fact, we have all seen people miss lifts at the top, especially in pressing movements involving the upper body. My point is the vast majority of presses that are missed are lost in the upper half of the range of movement.

Why should this be the case when we consider that in "machine theory," the top third of any movement should be easier due to muscle skeletal leverage advantages at that point? The answer is simple. When we approach the end of a given movement, certain muscle groups assume the role of primary movers. These

muscles may be smaller and less capable than the muscles that served as primary movers in the first two-thirds of the movement. Therefore, these smaller muscles, now thrust into the role of primary movers, have a great deal of stress to deal with and a limited capacity to handle it.

Consider the bench press, for example. At the beginning of the lift, i.e. off the chest, the primary movers are the pectoralis major and the deltoids. These are fairly large muscles with great potentials. Towards the end of the lift, i.e. upper third, there is a shift to the triceps as the primary movers. At this point in the lift, the pecs and delts have relatively little leverage. So the burden of completing the movement is left to a relatively small muscle group, the triceps. The triceps in no way compares potential-wise to the pec and delt group, and therefore a lifter often struggles in the final stages of the bench press.

Bearing this in mind, how can the companies who produce these variable resistance devices justify the application of this principle to all their machines? I submit that they cannot. Granted, the principle of variable resistance may have valid application with regard to some exercises, but this same principle has its limitations, and these limitations should be explored.

Considering the cost/effectiveness ratio of devices that may not be designed on universally justifiable principles, there comes a question of procurement desirability. Why should anyone buy a device founded on a principle which is neither universally applicable nor fundamentally accepted? My criticism applies directly to those manufacturers who use variable resistance devices in *all* their products.

The main thing to remember when trying to improve strength is, while theory is fine, practical application is everything. Men like Anderson, Alexeev, Rigert, Cole and Rheinhout, trained principally with methods that had sound, practical application. These men became among the strongest on earth and are universally accepted as such. Coincidentally, all the above men became awesomely strong using *free weights*—not machines.

ROUTINES

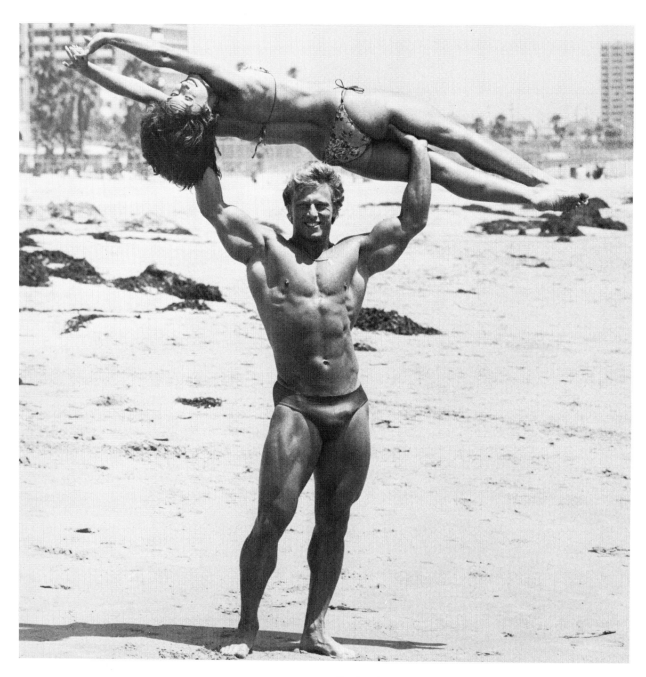

"Strive for excellence, exceed yourself, love your friend, speak the truth, practice fidelity and honor your father and mother. These principles will help you master yourself, make you strong, give you hope and put you on a path to greatness."

—Joe Weider
Trainer of Champions

Beginner's Bodybuilding Training

by Andreas Cahling

You have made your big decision: You are going to become a bodybuilder. You have read your first copy of *Muscle & Fitness* or flipped out over the green-tinted muscles of the Incredible Hulk. Every great bodybuilder was once a beginner like you. He was innocent. He didn't know any more than you do. He had to learn. If he was lucky, he got started right.

Beginners are wide-eyed and impressionable. They are fragile creatures who truly believe that one day they will be Mr. Universe or Mr. Olympia. The beauty of that dream is that it is within reach if they understand the value of persistence.

First of all, every beginner should realize that no quality physique has ever been built in less than three or four years. It takes time and persistence. The young guy who reconciles to the long apprenticeship will have an advantage. Invariably he will be the one who succeeds regardless of his potential. Success does not end with success. People like Ed Corney, 45, and Tony Emmott, 40, continue to improve. Frank Zane, 38, who won the Mr. Olympia title three times, continues to train and improve. Says he: "I continue to train and compete because I know I can still get better every year."

Potential is a fixed quantity. The beginner's dazzling dream blinds him to his potential and his strong and weak points. As the months go by his vision will clear. He will get a better look at his skeletal structure and be better able to ascertain his muscle growth rate. Some revelations may hurt and frustrate. Others will excite him. His inner calf may be deficient, providing a long fight ahead. But those clavicles that always seemed bony and prominent, may also be long, and will be a good base for developing powerful, broad shoulders.

All beginners must follow the same type of program for anywhere from six weeks to four months. The rate of progress depends on the kind of shape you are in when you begin bodybuilding. If you have been active in sports, you will be able to work harder initially. If you have been inactive physically, the weights will feel clumsy and you will tire sooner.

Age has little bearing on beginning bodybuilders. Anyone who has reached puberty (14–15 years of age) can expect good results. Before that age, results are not as fast. For the next 25 years you will have every chance to build a championship physique. If you start past the age of 40, you can still build an impressive body, but don't expect to win Mr. Olympia. I know a man who started bodybuilding training at the age of 56, and now at 63 he has a fine physique.

As a beginner you should train at least three, and no more than four, days a week. If you train three days a week, always separate the workouts by a day of rest. For example, you can train Monday, Wednesday and Friday, or Tuesday, Thursday and Saturday, whatever is convenient.

Then start:

1. Situps: 1 X 20–50
2. Calf Machine: 3 X 15–29 (40%)
3. Parallel Squat: 3 X 10–15 (35%)
4. Bent Row: 3 X 8–12 (30%)
5. Upright Row: 3 X 8–12 (25%)
6. Bench Press: 3 X 8–12 (30%)
7. Military Press: 3 X 8–12 (25%)
8. Barbell Curl: 3 X 8–12 (25%)
9. Lying Triceps Extension: 3 X 8–12 (25%)
10. Wrist Curl: 3 X 15–20 (20%)

The numbers, 3 X 8–12, mean three sets of eight to 12 repetitions. A repetition ("rep") is one complete movement of any exercise. A set is a group of reps. Eight consecutive reps would be called a set of eight.

Between sets we usually rest about 60 seconds. Perform all the required sets of each exercise before moving on to the next one.

During the first two weeks you should do only one set of each exercise, the third week two sets, and the sixth week three sets. Lifting weights is heavier exercise than anything you have ever done, so it is advisable to break in gradually. If you rush it, your muscles will get abysmally sore. You will probably become mildly sore anyway, a condition that soon disappears as your body adapts to the heavier work. Should you become uncomfortably sore, take a hot bath.

The percentages listed after the sets and reps refer to suggested starting weights related to the percentage of your bodyweight. For example, in the parallel squat a 150-pound man would start out using 50 to 55 pounds, which is 35 percent of his bodyweight.

These recommended poundages may seem a little light to some, heavier to others. It will be up to you to adjust the poundages to match your capability. If you can do the required repetitions with ease, increase the resistance by five or 10 pounds for the next workout. If it is a strain to do the required reps, decrease the resistance by five or 10 pounds.

You will notice that I have listed a range of repetitions for each exercise with two guide numbers, one low, one high. For example: Parallel Squat: 3 X 10–15 (35%) means you may use 50 pounds for 10 reps to start, then with each successive workout you will do an additional rep until you are doing 15 reps six workouts after you have started. Once you have reached 15 reps with 50 pounds, add weight and drop your reps back down to the lower guide number, e.g. 55 X 10 reps, and begin working up again.

Muscles grow larger and stronger in response to progressively increased resistance, so you should always endeavor to lift heavier and heavier weights. One additional rep is the minimum you should attempt, because many times you will be able to add more. Just be sure you don't add weight by "cheating" up the barbell through such actions as a knee kick or back bend. Strict form is essential for beginners.

When you can comfortably do three sets of each exercise, progressively do additional sets until you are doing five sets of each exercise. Add the sets at a rate of one new set each workout on one exercise only. In other words, after you have reached three sets on each exercise, it will take an additional nine workouts to bring you up to four sets per exercise (situps

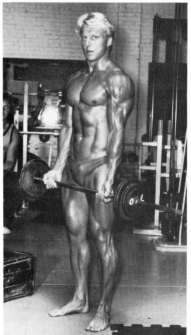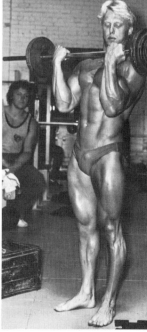

BARBELL CURL—Stand erect with a shoulder-width reverse grip on the bar. Move the barbell in a semicircle to your chin, keeping your upper arms motionless. Lower and repeat for full biceps growth.

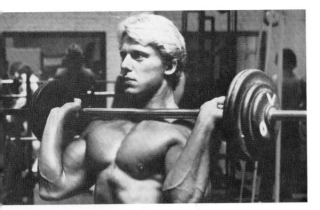

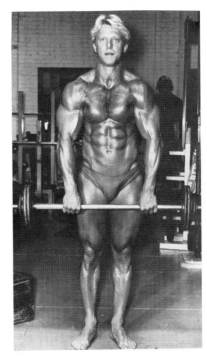

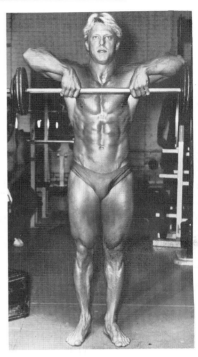

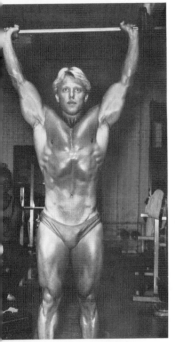

UPRIGHT ROW—Pull the barbell smoothly from your thighs to chin level, tense at the top, lower and repeat. Be sure to lower the bar as slowly as you raise it. I like this movement for my shoulders and upper back.

MILITARY PRESS—Stand erect with the barbell at your shoulders and take a grip slightly wider than shoulder width. Push the barbell slowly to arms' length directly ahead. Lower and repeat. This is an excellent shoulder excercise.

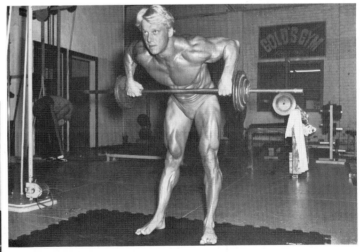

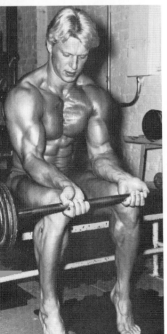

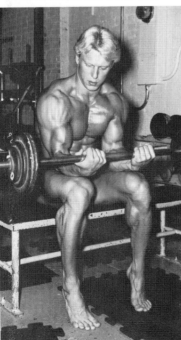

BENT ROW—To develop back width and thickness, bend over to the position illustrated and pull the barbell from straight arms' length to the chest, as if rowing a boat.

WRIST CURL—Maintaining the position shown, slowly flex and extend your wrist. Get a full range of motion and do high repetions. This works your forearms.

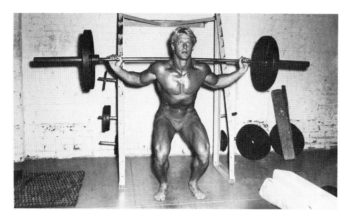

SQUAT—With a barbell behind your neck, keep your head up and squat down until your thighs reach an imaginary line parallel to the floor. Come erect and repeat. Your thighs will get a great workout from Squats.

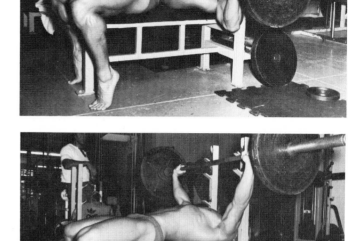

BENCH PRESS—Lying on your back, press a barbell straight up, then let it descend. Be sure you force your upper arms straight out to the sides as you press the barbell. This works your chest muscles.

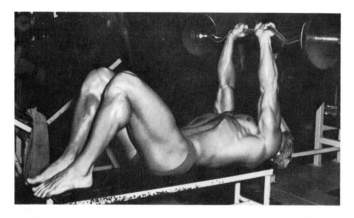

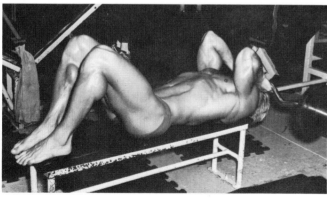

LYING TRICEPS EXTENSION—Start with an EZ-curl bar at straight arms' length. Bend your elbows and lower the weight in a semicircle to your forehead. Keep your upper arms still at all times to fully work your triceps.

are excluded), and finally nine more workouts to bring you up to five sets per exercise.

For optimum results you must get sufficient rest and follow a proper diet. Sleep requirements vary with individuals, but eight hours of good sound sleep each night is a realistic guide. A short nap or rest at some time during the day is worthwhile.

Eat at least three good meals per day, plus a quality snack or two. Stay away from sugar and flour products, fried foods, alcohol and processed foods like potato chips and TV dinners. Instead, eat a balanced diet of fresh foods from these three major groups:

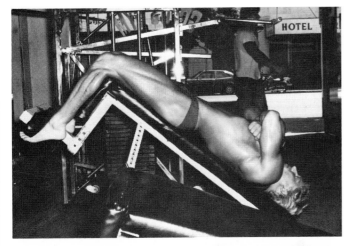

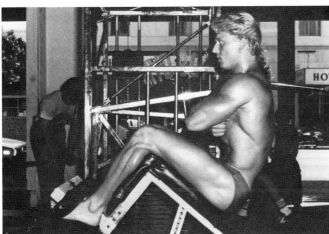

Proteins: Fish, poultry, milk, eggs, etc.
Fruit: Apples, oranges, grapefruit, peaches, etc.
Vegetables and salads: Beans, greens, carrots, etc.

It would also be a good idea to take vitamin and mineral supplements as insurance against progress-slowing nutritional deficiencies. At a minimum I would recommend Weider's Multi-Vitamin Mineral "100" and Protozyme Tabs (which aid in thoroughly digesting the food you eat). If you can afford it, also get some High-Potency B-Complex Caps, Sugar Potency Vitamin C, Liver Concentrate and Supreme E Caps. If you are underweight, and want to gain quickly, use a "Crash Weight" Plan as advertised in *Muscle & Fitness.*

These are the raw materials that you need to get started as a beginning bodybuilder. Train hard and train consistently—don't skip a workout! Be persistent and a physique trophy may be within closer reach than you think.

INCLINE SITUPS—To sharpen your abs, I recommend all variations of the Situp. The pictures are self-explanatory. Just be sure on all Situps to keep your knees bent. This takes strain off the lower back.

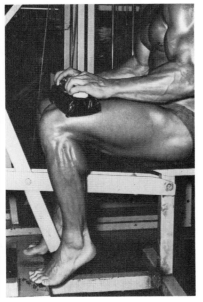

SEATED CALF MACHINE—After wedging your knees under the padded bar, move your heels up and down as far as possible. Try to do one set with more weight on your big toe. This develops the calf muscles.

actually crave a harder workout.

There are three basic ways to increase training intensity:

1. Increase the exercise poundage
2. Increase the sets and/or reps
3. Decrease the time it takes to do a particular amount of work

Until contest time, play with the first two variables, constantly trying to use heavier and heavier weights, always in strict form. As the contest nears, decrease training time. This is an advanced technique reserved for advanced bodybuilders who have competition in mind.

For the intermediate bodybuilder, increasing training intensity means increasing the number of sets—to as many as 10 per body part—and also increasing the exercise weights. Slowly and systematically add sets to your workout. Haste makes waste. As a general rule, you can safely add about one set per body part every two weeks.

Once you are doing six or more sets per body part, it would be a good idea to switch over to a four-day split routine, working half your body on Monday and Thursday, the other half on Tuesday and Friday. This method shortens each workout and enables you to intensify training for each muscle group.

Most intermediates can use the four-day split for a year or more. Indeed, many excellent bodybuilders train four days per week during the off-season and use a six-day split four to six weeks prior to an important competition. If you feel you are able to train six days a week after a year or so, try one of the following six-day split routines:

Training each body part two times per week
    Mon–Thurs—Chest, back
    Tues–Fri—Shoulders, arms
    Wed–Sat—Thighs
    Daily—Calves, abs

Training each body part three times per week
    Mon–Wed–Fri—Chest, shoulders,
      triceps, forearms
    Tues–Thurs–Sat—Thighs, back, biceps
    Daily—Calves, abs

The ultimate split routine—which is so demanding it can be used only by the champions of the sport—is the double split. When you get to that level, you can train twice per day, doing only one or two body parts per workout.

By the time you are doing 10 sets per body part, you will be ready for such advanced training principles as Supersets, Negative Reps and Forced Reps. It may take as long as a year to reach this level, and it should commence in the last 10% of your intermediate training. This is where you generate the final bit of momentum that will carry you into the advanced level and toward your first contest, if that is your goal.

Supersets, Negative Reps and Forced Reps should be fully understood, and back issues of *Muscle & Fitness* magazine carry complete information about these methods. So save your magazines, and what you don't have you can borrow from your buddies.

Briefly, supersets consist of doing two exercises together—no rest between them—and then resting for a minute or two. Contest bodybuilders often do supersets within a muscle group, e.g. Preacher Curls and Seated Dumbbell Curls as a superset for biceps. But intermediates should superset only antagonistic muscle groups, like biceps-triceps, chest-back, etc.

Forced reps are done at the end of a set when a training partner helps you force out a rep or two more than you could normally do. By pushing past the point of normal muscle failure in this manner, you can stimulate faster growth.

Negative reps require a training partner or two who will lift up the weight for you so you can lower it slowly. This is called *eccentric contraction*, and exercise physiologists have recently shown it's highly beneficial in stimulating muscle growth.

As you move into these higher training levels, you will be making the most of your instinctive training knowledge. Keep written notes on every workout. Monitor everything: fatigue, diet, appetite, pump, hardness, growth, energy level, irritability, muscle ache, soundness of sleep, and any other manifestation of your body or mind as they react to the rigors of training.

You will have a computer full of information and you'll be able to get in touch with your body, your training techniques, how you felt, etc. at any given point since you started pumping iron. In that way, you can fully control and literally predict your progress.

Advanced Training

by Andreas Cahling

Now you have arrived at the advanced level of training. You have paid your dues as an intermediate. Naivety has given way to reality. You dream less of greatness and more about tomorrow's workout. You bargain for more body weight, but usually settle for the slightest improvement in muscular shape, density and definition. You barely remember the good old days when you could gain a pound of muscle a month. You have come to realize that great size isn't everything.

Robby Robinson has made this crystal clear. "Size is fantastic, and all of the foremost bodybuilders are huge, but when everyone is as big as the next guy, it takes something more. That something more is fine muscular detail—deep separations between the major muscle masses, plus fine little striations within each of these masses."

Bodybuilders aren't just born with these striations. I'm sure you've seen bodybuilders with striations like cat claw marks across their pecs. To some extent this is a function of diet—you have to be low in body fat for muscle to show through your skin—but it's more a result of maximum training intensity and the use of the Weider advanced training principles.

Advanced training is a refinement of what you learned as an intermediate bodybuilder:

1. Continually increasing intensity of training;

2. Expanded use of the Weider principles of forced reps, cheating and continuous tension;

3. Continuing use of basic exercises to maintain muscle mass and build additional shape;

4. Specialization on existing weak areas through increasing machine training;

5. Cycle training; and

6. Visualization technique.

Continuous tension is probably a contest bodybuilder's best weapon. It brings out the striations Robinson was referring to earlier. Not only should you feel the weight through its entire range of motion by doing slow and controlled reps, but you should also build additional tension into the muscle by tensing the muscles antagonistic to those doing the work. For example, on Concentration Curls, you should make the weight "heavier" by contracting the triceps as you are putting maximum tension into the biceps.

While continuous tension and isolation exercises like Concentration Curls are valuable refinements, it would be folly to neglect basic exercises. The muscle-mass-conscious bodybuilders like the Squat, Bench Press and Bent-Over Rowing motion. If you neglect these exercises, you'll end up with plenty of muscular detail, but no appreciable muscle mass.

I would suggest that you always—even in pre-contest training—do at least one basic exercise per body part. Then you can also do two to four isolation movements to shape and striate the muscles. If you're doing delts, then start with a few heavy sets of Presses Behind The Neck for mass. After that you can do several sets each of Bent Laterals, Front Laterals and Cable Side Laterals for the finished look that it takes to win contests.

Tying in with the use of basic exercises is the Weider Cheating Principle. I haven't mentioned cheating until this advanced stage of training, since it takes a very intelligent bodybuilder to use cheating correctly. Too many novices cheat to remove stress from a muscle, when cheating should actually be used to place *more* stress on the muscle group being worked.

For example, Cheating Curls are great for the biceps, but not if you cheat merely to get a heavy weight up and then sloppily lower it. The slight cheating swing should just be used to get a heavy weight started up; after this point, biceps strength finishes the curl. On the way down, the curl should be forcefully resisted which puts even more stress on your biceps.

In general, I favor cheating only toward the end of a hard set, not on every rep of a full set. If you can go one or two reps past your usual failure point by cheating, you'll experience the ecstasy of full-growth stimulation.

When you are pushing to the limits of your strength and endurance in every workout, you will experience steady muscle growth. But the only way you'll be able to push this hard is to get your mind totally into your workouts. You must use every little mental trick at your command if you want to cross the threshold between being an average bodybuilder and an Olympian.

One mental technique I use in all of my training is *visualization*. It's fully explained in my Viking Power Training Secrets course, but I think I can describe it concisely for this short article.

Visualization takes advantage of a psychological principle called *self-actualization*. What literally happens is that your subconscious mind coldly and calculatedly makes choices to make you become what you want to be in life. If your life's goal is to be a concert pianist, you subconsciously will make the choices you need to make to reach this particular goal.

In bodybuilding, we can program our minds to achieve tremendous physical goals. When I have an important competition coming up, I will

visualize myself, for 10–15 minutes several times per day, as I plan to be on the day of the contest. I give myself a generous helping of muscle mass, proportions, striations, tan, posing technique, charisma and general appearance when I do this visualization.

If I can make all of these things real to myself several times per day, my subconscious mind will be correctly programmed to bring me to contest shape exactly as I've visualized it and at the correct time. Believe me, it's worked for me several times.

Once your mind has been programmed, everything comes easier. It's easier to diet, you sleep better, you train harder and you don't even mind spending boring hours in the sun. It's all so easy, because your subconscious mind is taking a load off your conscious mind by making all the decisions. Give this technique a try.

The final advanced technique I'd like to mention is *cycle training*. Very simply, it involves two different philosophies, one for pre-contest and one for off-season training. If you read *Muscle & Fitness* carefully each month, you'll know all you need to know about peaking for a

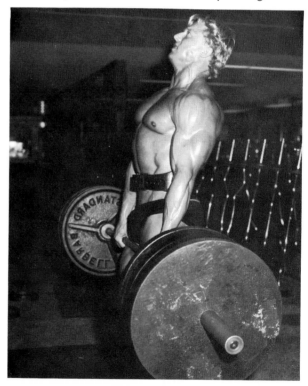

"Constantly increasing the intensity of training, to build mass and razor sharp striations, without burning out in the process, is one of the secrets of advanced training."

—Andreas Cahling

competition, so concentrate on working toward a more productive off-season cycle.

In my off-season cycle, I have two goals: to bring up a weak point or two, and to add general overall muscle mass. To accomplish these aspirations, I tend to train heavier overall, for mass, and rearrange my workouts to put more time on a weakness and less on my stronger areas. If you can just maintain a strong point while bringing up a weak one, you'll go into the pre-contest training phase miles ahead of where you were the last time.

So you should begin using cycle training and entering contests. Put at least three months into each building cycle and 6–8 weeks into each contest preparation phase. By alternating the two, you will gradually get bigger and more proportionate, with contest-winning muscular detail. With that combination, there's no way you can lose!

Lou Ferrigno:
Working to Break the 60-Inch Chest Barrier

by Lou Ferrigno
with Bill Reynolds

You can't lie to 50 million people!

On a recent episode of the Mike Douglas Show, Mike brought out a tape measure to see how big around I was in a few selected areas. I welcomed the opportunity to be measured before a national TV audience.

My upper arms were 22 3/4 inches cold, my chest a bit over 56 cold and relaxed. So I think you can believe me when I tell you that my pumped biceps measurement is now 23 1/2 and my chest expanded and pumped is 59 inches at 275 pounds body weight.

That 59-inch chest measurement has me fired up to burst past the 60-inch barrier. That's no-man's land. There's never been a bodybuilder with a chest over 60 inches. So you can see why I'm so up for crossing the threshold.

Still, I'm not going for 60 just for the sake of hitting 60. A measurement like that is sure death to a bodybuilder if it's out of proportion to the rest of his body. The way I'm training now will cause my chest to keep growing, but I have to be careful that my arms, delts, back and legs go up at the same rate as my chest. Proportion is the whole ball game at the Olympian level, and I gotta play by the rules.

Don't get the idea that I was born with a big chest. When I first started bodybuilding, it was only 40 inches, and by then I was already almost six feet tall. My chest and legs have always been the slowest to develop, so I've had to work exceptionally hard on my rib cage and pectorals. With hard work, however, my chest has gradually inched up and developed over the years.

Fully expanding the rib cage is one essential factor in developing an impressive chest. This is particularly important in the early stages of bodybuilding, since the rib box is the foundation on which you build your whole torso. To develop your chest, back and shoulders to their ultimate potential, you have to fully expand your rib cage.

Chest expansion comes from a combination of breath-stimulating and chest-stretching movements. I have always done heavy leg work to stimulate breathing and push my ribs outward. Dumbbell Pullovers, while lying across a bench, are my favorite stretching exercise. Do five sets of Squats and three sets of Pullovers, hitting 12–20 reps on each set. If you go too high on the reps, your exercise weights will be excessively light.

On the Pullovers, I hold a heavy dumbbell in both hands and rest my shoulders and upper back across a flat bench. My elbows are always slightly bent, since that tends to give me a better stretch, and it takes pressure off my elbows. At

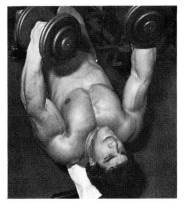
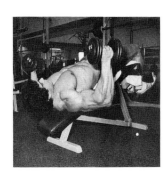
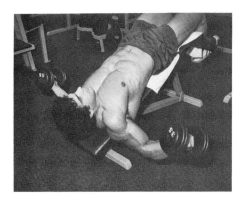

START/"Decline Flyes give me a clean line around the lower and outer pectorals."/FINISH

the low point of the movement I also drop my hips as low as possible, because that also encourages a greater stretching of the rib cage. And finally, I never bring the dumbbell all the way back up above my chest. It only goes back to a point over my forehead, which keeps tension on the chest throughout the set.

It will take at least a year of steady effort to enlarge the rib box. The results, however, are well worth the effort, and you'll probably continue to do the Pullovers for life. I still do them, and my rib cage continues to grow in volume.

The pectorals are much easier to build. The secret is to hit them from all angles. You also have to use the basic exercises—Bench Presses, Incline Presses, Decline Presses and Parallel Bar Dips. These are the heavy movements that pack muscle on your chest. Flyes, Crossovers and Peck Deck work are for shaping and striating the pecs, and you'll find that those exercises do little to enhance muscle mass.

It's an absolute must to do Bench Presses in every chest workout. They hit the whole pectoral mass, as well as the shoulders, triceps and lats. They pack power into your upper body like no other exercise. Indeed, you could get a tremendous full body workout for both strength and development on just Squats, Benches and Bent Rows.

Inclines are for the upper chest, and Declines and Dips hit primarily the lower and outer edges of your pectorals. On the heavy pressing movements, a lot of bodybuilders use an excessively wide grip. My grip for all of my presses is only slightly wider than shoulder width. That gives me both a better stretch at the bottom and a tighter contraction at the top of the movement.

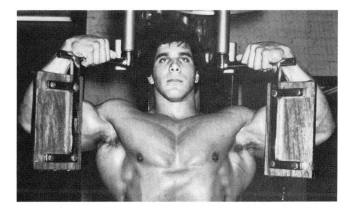

START/"I use the Peck Deck as an alternative to Flyes."
"Actually, I'm too big to use the machine properly."
/FINISH

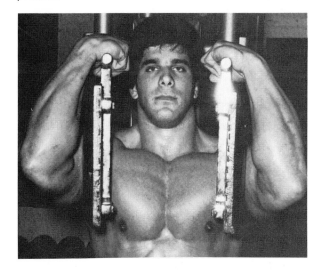

At times I'll do angled presses with dumbbells. The dumbbells let you stretch lower at the bottom, since there's no bar to run into the chest before the hands reach the lowest possible position. This is a good thing prior to a contest when you're trying for more shape and

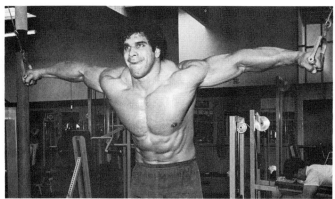

START/"Cable Crossovers are my favorite pre-contest pectoral movement, because they really striate my pecs."

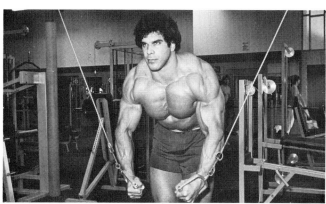

"It's important to crunch hard at the bottom of the movement."/FINISH

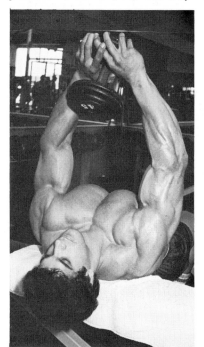

START/"Cross-Bench Pullovers expand my rib cage . . ."

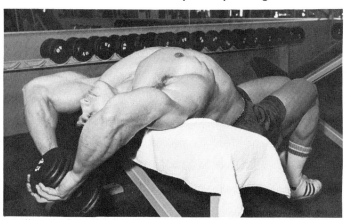

". . . and tie the lats, pecs and serratus together."/FINISH

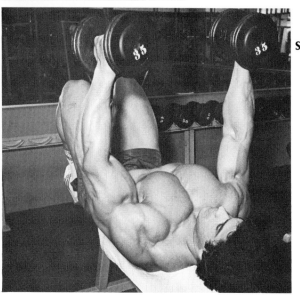

START/"Flyes are basic pec-shaping exercises."

"They're second only to the bench press." /FINISH

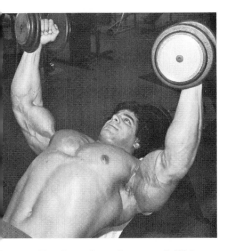

TART/"Incline Flyes shape and fill in he upper pectorals."

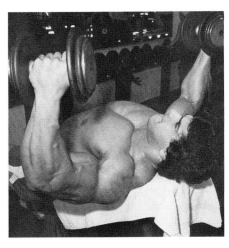

MIDPOINT/"Be sure to force your elbows back as you lower the weight."

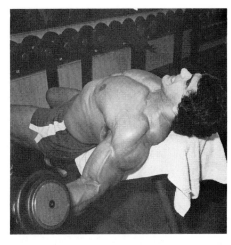

FINISH/"You should also go as low as possible on each repetition."

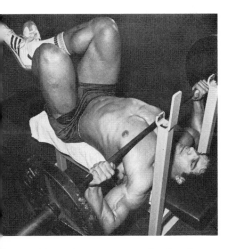

TART/"Bench Presses are absolutely he most important chest movement."

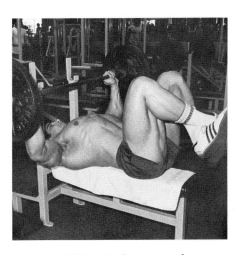

MIDPOINT/"Again, be sure to keep your elbows back for direct pec stimulation."

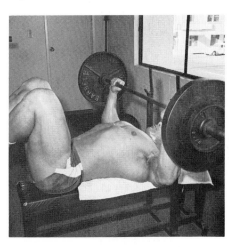

FINISH/"Hold the finish position for a second and tense your pecs hard."

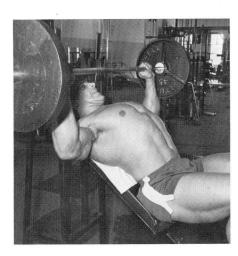

MIDPOINT/"Incline Presses are the basic upper excercise."

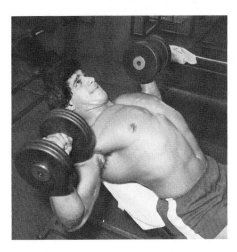

START/"You can some times switch over to Dumbell Inclines."

muscularity. But for pure mass, I get far more out of the barbell pressing exercises.

The key to effectively using the various types of Flye exercises is to get a full stretch and to build a lot of tension into the muscles during the movement. When I'm after striations just before a contest, I really work the Pulley Crossovers hard, since that exercise enables me to put maximum tension on my pecs.

Prior to a contest, I'll tense my chest a lot between sets. I'll also do plenty of posing at home at night. Joe Weider showed me how to use these tension techniques, and I've found them to be invaluable for etching in the finest lines all over my body before a show.

Every week I receive hundreds of letters asking for training routines. It should be obvious that it's impossible for me to respond to such a massive number of requests, so I'd like to take this opportunity to give you four graduated chest workouts. One of them will be appropriate for you, and within a year or so you could probably work up through all four.

Beginners should do five or six sets of Bench Presses right from the beginning. Do only the Benches, but work them hard. Do the first set with a moderate weight for 12 reps. Add some weight—say, 10–20 pounds—and do 10 reps. Successively add weight and drop the reps over an 8-7-6-5 range. Be sure that the last set of five reps is at your maximum, and once you can do the full five reps, add 5-10 pounds to every set for your next workout.

Intermediate bodybuilders—those with 3–6 months of steady training behind them—should stick to the Bench Presses and add a shaping movement like Flyes. A little later an intermediate can also include the Pullovers I mentioned earlier. Intermediates should do something in the neighborhood of 8–12 total sets in their chest routine.

Advanced bodybuilders can do four different exercises and about five sets for each chest movement. At the end of the intermediate phase, or the beginning of the advanced phase, one should start putting priority on weaknesses, such as the upper chest or the inner edges of the pectorals. Here's a good advanced routine:

1. Bench Press: 6 X 5–12
2. Incline Press: 5 X 6–10
3. Flyes: 5 X 10
4. Pullovers: 4 X 15–20

The above routine is basically what I do in regular training. If I was getting ready for the Olympia, however, I'd intensify my workouts to this level:

1. Bench Press: 5 X 6–10
2. Incline Press: 5 X 6–10
3. Decline Press: 5 X 6–10
4. Flyes: 5 X 10–12
5. Cross-Bench Pullovers: 3 X 15,
        supersetted with . . .
6. Cable Crossovers: 3 X 10–15

Because my chest responds slowly, I use the Weider Muscle Priority Principle, training my chest early in my workout when my energy and training drive are greatest. Lately I've been doing chest, shoulders and triceps together on Mondays and Thursdays. On Tuesdays-Fridays I do back and biceps, and on Wednesdays-Saturdays I train my thighs. I do some abdominal and calf work daily.

I do forced reps for all of my body parts, but I think a lot of guys use forced reps incorrectly. They do one very hard forced rep and quit. I'd prefer to do my full set, have my partner support 20–25% of the weight and then do 2-3 forced reps with him pulling up to help me. You can't let yourself get too fatigued from a single set. If you do, your strength level will be too low for you to do justice to the rest of the workout.

The final tip I'll leave you with involves the role of my mind in my bodybuilding formula. Overall, I'd say that diet is about 60% and training 40% of the battle in bodybuilding, but the mind is the glue that holds this whole structure together. Without the mind, training and diet both approach 0% effectiveness.

You have to concentrate. If you're after a pump, you have to think about that pump. I have to eat, sleep and think about bodybuilding. At the gym, I block out everything but my workout. I'll talk with someone only before or after a workout.

I spend a good 1-1½ hours psyching up before a workout. I think about what I have to train, what exercises I have to do, how I'm going to feel, etc. I have a cup of coffee and try to erase all negative thoughts from my mind. Then I go to the gym and put 100% into my workout.

A bodybuilder has to improve every year, or he'll never reach the top. Even though I'm involved in show business now, I am still putting 100% into my training. I want to be Mr. Olympia more than I've ever wanted anything in my life. I can only do one thing at a time, but one day I plan to come back to competitive bodybuilding and absolutely dominate the sport. You can bet on it!

My Definitive Biceps Workout

by Arnold Schwarzenegger
as told to Bill Reynolds

For almost as long as he can remember, biceps have been a high priority for Arnold Schwarzenegger, seven-time Mr. Olympia and winner of 12 world championships. "I think I have some good heredity for bodybuilding," Arnold said recently, "but I don't think it was the make-or-break factor for biceps. It's more important that when I was 10 years old, I was already flexing my arms every day.

"By the time I started bodybuilding at age 15, biceps were the most noticeable muscle group on my body, because that's what I had been flexing a lot. And my only arm work that first year was for biceps, because I didn't even know there was such a thing as triceps. We didn't have the magazines to read then—like people do over here—so I had little knowledge of training.

"Of course when you flex a muscle group so many thousands of times more than others, it is going to be better. By flexing my biceps so much, I'd learned to control them more completely. My mind was right there in my biceps when I flexed them, and I could gain great control of my biceps before I ever touched a weight. This mind-link ability then translated

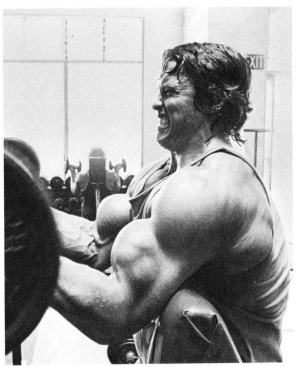

"Preacher Curls are particularly effective if you have an inherently short biceps."

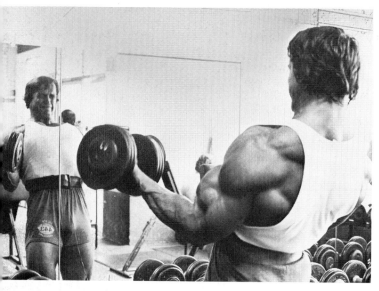

"The key on Dumbbell Curls is to fully supinate your hands as the weights go up."

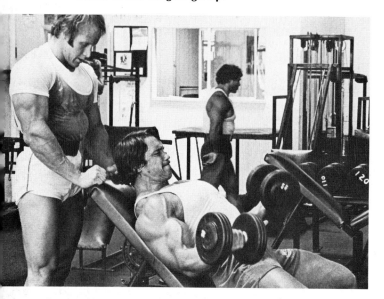

"Doing Curls on an incline bench forces you to do the movement strictly, thus stimulating phenominal growth."

into my bodybuilding when I began training with weights. When I did a curl, it felt special, because I could instantly sense blood rushing into the muscle.

"Because I adopted a certain favoritism toward the biceps at such an early age, they grew easily and got a little ahead of the rest of my body. But isn't the name of the game at the Olympian level total body balance? I was defeating myself by having such comparatively mind-blowing biceps because it threw my proportions out of balance. My triceps and forearms looked small in comparison.

"My decision on how to train toward better arm balance did not include any lessening of biceps workout intensity. Instead, the triceps caught up because I was always careful to do at least five more sets for triceps than biceps. The triceps are a potentially bigger mass than biceps, and the bigger a muscle the more sets you'll need to thoroughly train it.

"I kept my biceps training very hard but put more emphasis on triceps to bring them up. The name of the game was to get the right proportions and perfect symmetry. An intelligent bodybuilder will identify such weaknesses as I had in my early years and then work hard to bring these areas up to par. When he does this, he will eventually become a true champion. That is, of course, if he has certain potentials.

"While some have better growth rate potential than others, a more important heredity point is the shape of each bodybuilder's biceps. By being persistent, you can eventually build the size and quality needed to win titles, but if your biceps is naturally flat, it is extremely difficult to build an incredible peak on it.

"From the very first, I had a natural peak, which became accentuated as I trained. I was blessed with round, football-shaped biceps, while others—like Sergio Oliva and Larry Scott— had natural length and fullness but not a great peak. Heredity causes the peak, but it doesn't cause a person to have a 20- or 21-inch arm. That comes from hard training."

Listening to the Austrian Oak talk, one is quickly convinced that a powerful mind should be the base of every quarter inch of new muscle growth. "Throughout my bodybuilding career," Arnold recalls, "I was constantly playing tricks on my mind. This is why I began to think of my biceps as mountains, instead of flesh and blood. Thinking of my biceps as a mountain made my arms grow faster and bigger than if I'd seen them only as a muscle.

"When you think of biceps as merely a muscle, you subconsciously have a limit in your mind, which for biceps is something in the 20- or 21-inch area. When you limit yourself to that measurement, it is very hard to get to that level, and needless to say impossible to get past that measurement. But when you think about a mountain, there is no mental limit to biceps growth, and therefore you have a chance of going beyond normal mental barriers.

"This is almost like a psychic phenomenon of sport. They had the four-minute barrier in the mile run, for example, and nobody could beat that barrier, it seemed. But once Roger Bannister ran under 4:00, everyone seemed to be doing it. Four minutes was just a mental barrier, and once broken, it no longer existed.

"I didn't want to set up any barriers in my arm training, because many years ago 18 inches was an arm barrier, then 19, then 20, which Leroy Colbert finally broke. These obstacles—these limits—are placed on you not by your body, but by your mind. Thinking of mountains simply eliminated biceps barriers for me."

As Schwarzenegger was talking about arm barriers, I personally found it difficult to believe that he had spent much time taking measurements, since most of the champions I've interviewed relied on the mirror to evaluate progress. "It wasn't very often that I got out the tape, and that was usually when I was at my heaviest bodyweight. Then—at 245 to 250—my upper arm measurement was in excess of 22 inches cold.

"At times just before a competition, I would measure my arm merely to see how much it had dropped from the strict dieting and consequent bodyweight loss. Even then, it measured past 21 inches cold. Otherwise, I didn't measure much, because I was at a stage of concentrating on perfection rather than size. I measured my arms much more at earlier stages, when I was 19 or 20, going after pure size. Then I could see size increases every week."

During his "growing boy" days—when he was winning his first Mr. Universe title at 19 years of age—Arnold trained much differently than in his later competitive years. "For biceps," he remembers, "I was always using the basic exercises—barbell curls, dumbbell curls—with heavy weights. In most workouts, we would go up to 225 pounds in the barbell curl.

"This was a pretty strict movement, because I remember at the time doing cheating curls with 275 for three or four reps. With 225, I would rest each repetition on my thighs for a moment, inhale and exhale, and then pull it up again, instead of just throwing the bar up and down.

"On dumbbell curls, I was very careful to supinate my hands fully as I curled the weights up. I'm sure this supination movement is largely responsible for the fullness and peak I eventually attained for each biceps. The biceps come into play quite strongly to supinate your hands, as well as to flex the arm. This little twist gave me the separation, the brachialis development and the lower biceps thickness.

"So what is supination? I'm sure that many *Muscle & Fitness* readers are unfamiliar with this term, so perhaps I should explain it. If you are

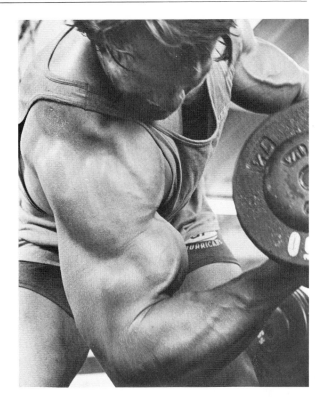

"To peak the biceps, nothing beats Concentration Curls. Note that I prefer doing this exercise with my elbow free from my body."

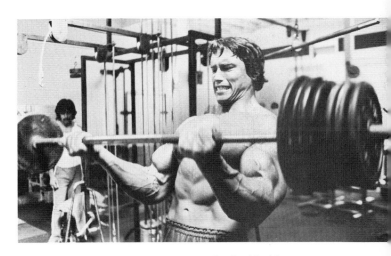

"Barbell Curls are the most basic and valuable biceps movement. Don't be afraid to pile on plates, but not at the expense of strict excercise form."

doing curls with two dumbbells and supinating correctly, your palms will begin by facing directly toward each other when your arms are straight down at your sides.

"From there, with your arms still straight, rotate your thumbs toward each other to fully stretch your biceps. Then begin simultaneously curling the bells up and rotating your thumbs in the opposite direction—out away from each other—as the weight goes up. At the completion point, your arms should be fully flexed and your hands turned out as far as humanly possible. This turning out of the hands and wrists is the supination movement.

"When I did these curls correctly, there was always a stabbing sort of pain in my biceps at the top, a reassurance that I had fully contracted the muscles. I could only get this sensation when concentrating well, however. If my mind was wandering, I'd lose this flexing sensation. I'd feel like there was another inch of movement to go, but it just wouldn't come. That's when I knew my mind would need to be forced back to the task at hand.

"An average training program back in Munich would include barbell curls, dumbbell curls (seated or standing), preacher bench curls and concentration curls. Keep in mind, though, that the way I trained changed a lot of times, because I'd always try to shock the muscles. Toward this end, I'd do no typical number of sets or reps. I recall days when my training partners and I would do 20 extremely heavy sets of biceps work, with only four or five reps each set. Another day—maybe only two days later—we would do 10 more sets, 15 reps each, using a lighter weight.

"This *shocking method* was extremely important to my training. Your muscles tend to become complacent and resist growth if you are constantly doing the same workout for them. But if you try all different types of training methods, exercise weights, set-rep combinations and training tempos, you keep the muscles off balance. They sort of say to themselves, 'Wow, there's a new thing here. He just did 10 sets of 20 reps, and the next workout he'll do 20 sets of five reps. I'll never get used to this. I can never build up a resistance to the training, so I guess I'll have to grow!'

"If you need this variety in training—and I did—it can be a definite advantage for you to include it in your routines. I felt that I needed variety in order to maintain excitement in my training, and also to make the muscle respond. I believed that if I trained for two weeks exactly the same way—the same sets, same reps, etc.— the muscle would get too used to this and build up a resistance to a set type of workout. Therefore, it would cease to respond.

"This could be the same for almost everyone, but it depends on the mental makeup of each individual bodybuilder. Some feel more comfortable when sticking to the same routine six months or a year at a time. If that works, then it's better for you and you should stick with it. I never try to tell anyone that my way is the only way, because everyone is an individual, with individual exercise and nutrition requirements."

In the summer of 1975—before he went to South Africa for his sixth Mr. Olympia win— Arnold was still training with a good deal of variety, but was doing less sets than a few years previously. "By then I could train with more intensity," Schwarzenegger reveals, "and I also didn't want to exaggerate my biceps and throw off my proportions.

"At that point I might have done three exercises—typically barbell curls, dumbbell curls and concentration curls—with four sets of six to 10 reps on each. Almost always, I would use a 'stripping method' for the barbell and dumbbell curls. This consisted of three sets within each set of curls, each done with a quick weight reduction. In other words, I would do several reps with a heavy barbell, have some plates stripped off while I took a short rest pause. Immediately after the plates were off, I would do a few more reps, strip more plates, and finally force out a final few, very hard repetitions.

"As I was working out, I would do each set until I couldn't do any more repetitions. Then I would put the weight down for a few seconds and open and close my fingers to relax. Almost immediately, I would pick up the weight again and do another two or three repetitions very slowly. During the set, there was a sensation of deep burning, as well as an extreme fullness in the arm. My arms were so pumped—they felt so great—when I finally stopped. The feeling put me on an instant high!

"I would almost always use a full, strict movement for biceps, except sometimes at the end of a set. I would do some burns from the bottom to lengthen the biceps. One thing that never changed was the tempo of the curls in each set.

"The weight would be raised slowly, and then lowered even more slowly, so I could feel resistance over the full range of motion. I'd say that I lowered the weight about 10 percent slower than I raised it, because we can get as much development from the downward segment of the movement as from the upward part, *if* we resist the weight as it is lowered."

Those who have seen the "Pumping Iron" film probably noticed how much posing the Oak did after training each body part. "I always tried to flex the biceps in various positions after working out. The problem with a lot of guys is that they only flex their biceps in one position—in a front double biceps shot. But then the biceps tends not to look good from the back, in a side chest shot or in a most muscular pose.

"I'd flex my arms in every possible position and tried to hold the flex as long as possible. This way my biceps—and other muscle groups, as well—would become used to the various postures I would need to hold at a prejudging, when poses must occasionally be held for relatively long periods of time.

"Another important thing is that I would pronate my hands (the opposite rotation to the supination already discussed, ed.) and straighten my arms between sets to fully stretch the biceps. This allowed blood to flow freely through my arms, flushing out waste products and bringing in a fresh supply of oxygen for the next set. Far too many bodybuilders tend to walk around the gym with their arms bent and biceps half contracted after a set. That closes down the arteries, so you need to concentrate on stretching. It really helped me."

Since bodybuilders of all experience levels read *Muscle & Fitness* magazine, I wanted to elicit Arnold's training advice for beginners and intermediates, as well as for advanced men. "For beginners, I'd simply advise doing five sets of barbell curls and five sets of dumbbell curls, doing ten total sets of eight to 12 repetitions. Concentrate on a strict movement, and try to gain some strength. Experiment with different curling arcs, until you find the one that puts maximum resistance on your biceps.

"Curling a weight strictly—like I've already described—is a difficult movement to make correctly, and I've rarely seen anyone take the time to learn to curl right. Even the most advanced bodybuilders seem to curl the easiest way possible, instead of the hard, correct way.

"When a bodybuilder does the movement poorly—when he just swings the weight up any way he can get it to his shoulders—it's usually because the barbell or dumbbells he picked are too heavy. So he swings, hunches or horses the weight up. He may be using the wrong curling arc, too. It's letting the muscle find the easiest groove to get the weight to the top, but the bottom line isn't merely to get the barbell or dumbbells up to your shoulders. It is to put full resistance on your biceps."

Intermediates? "By the time you've been training a year or so, I'd look at your biceps development and determine where you have weak points. Then I'd give you a tailored program to bring these weaker areas of your biceps up to par. Maybe you'll have no weak points, but after a year it will be easy to see them if they are there.

"You can see if the biceps are shorter—this was the case with Franco Columbu who consistently fought the problem of a short biceps. Of course, he finally triumphed, but only after years of intelligent training to overcome the weakness. If you have a short biceps, I'd recommend a lot of preacher curls, as well as some burns at the start of each curling movement. In time, this will fill in the gap between your biceps and the elbow.

"If you lack biceps fullness, do heavy dumbbell curls, being sure to fully supinate your wrists on every repetition. If you lack peak, stay totally away from barbell work, and do everything with dumbbells. Do plenty of concentration curls and dumbbell curls lying back on a high bench, like Reg Park used to do them. In this exercise, you get a great stretch.

"You have to get the biceps used to being fully stretched and curling up to a completely contracted position. That's what you get when you do dumbbell curls lying flat on your back. You stretch the biceps very hard, because your arm is going back, and then you get a peak contraction effect when you curl the bells up."

Any final advice for advanced bodybuilders? "The biggest post-intermediate level mistake is to burn the biceps out. The biceps is basically a small muscle group, and you can't do too much for it without overtraining. It's very small in relation to the thighs and back, so the muscle should be trained proportionately less.

"Generally speaking, a muscle twice as big as the biceps should be trained twice as much. I'd say that the upper limit for biceps would be 15 sets in a hard workout but I see all kinds of bodybuilders doing 25 to 30 sets on a regular basis.

"The number of days per week that the biceps should be trained is totally up to the individual. Indeed, this training frequency question can only be resolved by an individual bodybuilder after experimenting with both two-day and three-day training each week. I know champions who grow best on two times per week, and others who grow faster on three days per week. A few even make gains on some body parts training twice a week, and on others working out three days per week. Overall, I happen to be a three-times-per-week bodybuilder.

"Phase training is another important concept that advanced bodybuilders should master. This essentially consists of training differently in the off-season than prior to a contest. I'd personally concentrate primarily on my weak points for six to nine months of the off-season. Then as the next Olympia began to loom closer, I'd switch back to bombing the whole body.

"One year I'd emphasize forearms in the off-season, and the next it might be triceps or deltoids. Since biceps were a strong point from the beginning, I trained pretty much the same on them all year, merely experimenting with different movements in the off-season. If my biceps had been weak, however, I would have blasted the hell out of them during my noncompetitive phase."

In conclusion, Arnold Schwarzenegger summed up his ideas about what it takes to build a truly great set of biceps. "The important things are to do the movements correctly and concentrate your mind on making the biceps grow. Using the shocking method, the stripping method and all of the different training principles is also vital.

"Combine a very strong mind with optimum training and nutrition, and you can't help succeeding as a bodybuilder."

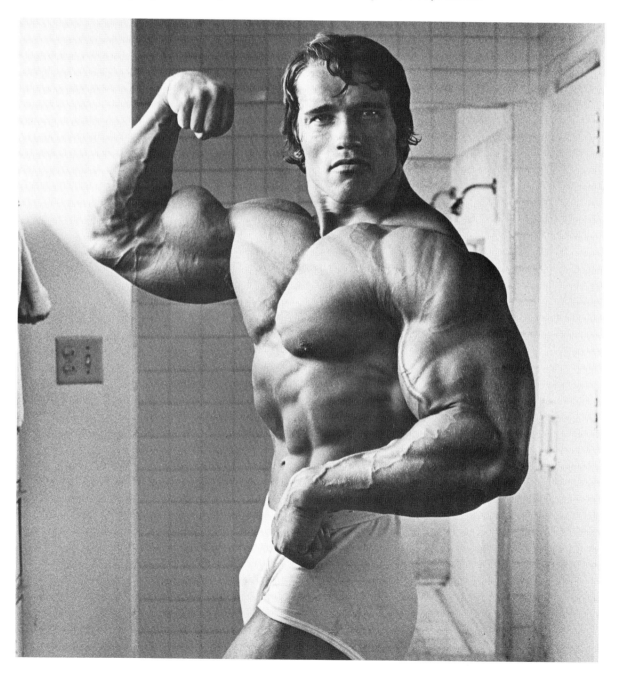

The Key to Big Arms

by Boyer Coe

Big arms—the goal of every bodybuilder. But when you say "big arms," the first thing that pops into most people's mind is a pair of well-developed biceps. Well, biceps are certainly an important part of the arm—you can't really have good arms without good biceps—but the muscles of the triceps on the back side of the arm actually account for most of the mass of the arm. The triceps, in fact, makes up two-thirds of the size of the arm. The size of the back head of the three-headed muscle gives the rear of the well-developed arm its powerful sweep.

So obviously a pair of well-developed triceps are an essential part of a pair of well-developed arms, and a triceps program is an indispensable part of the serious bodybuilder's training routine. It is a powerful muscle and can handle much hard direct work, as well as that which it gets in those movements involving pushing power, such as the military press and the bench press.

One of the best direct triceps exercises—and one that can be done by bodybuilders from the intermediate stage to the Mr. Olympia contender—is the triceps extension (sometimes called the triceps pushdown) done on the lat pulldown bar. This was the first triceps exercise I

learned, and I've stayed with it throughout my career; it is responsible for much of my triceps development, I'm sure.

When doing this extension movement, the spacing of the hands is very important. I recommend that it be a little narrower than shoulder width, with the elbows kept into the sides of the torso. The bar should be pushed down as far as possible for a good extension—until, in fact, you actually feel the elbows lock. Then allow the bar to come slowly and smoothly back up to the chest before you push it down again.

Avoid leaning into the movement, a bad habit that a lot of people let creep into this exercise. Actually, when you lean into the movement you are involving the deltoids directly. The idea of the exercise, of course, is to place the stress on the triceps—and the triceps alone. So keep your body straight up and down when you are doing these extensions. You may not be able to handle as much weight on the bar when you use this correct form, but it is more important that you isolate the triceps by doing the movement strictly.

Another triceps exercise I have used with good results is the lying triceps extension. This is done

79

from a lying position, as the name indicates, on a bench, using either a barbell or dumbbells for resistance. If a barbell is used, you might want to make it an E-Z curl bar; the variation this gives you on the grip will put added stress on the triceps. Here again it is quite important to keep the elbows in and pointed straight up and down throughout the exercise.

In the down—or stretch—position of the exercise, I allow the barbell to come down to touch the forehead. Then I push the bar back out so that the arms are straight ahead. I allow my head to hang sufficiently over the end of the bench so that the bar can come down as low as possible, allowing a full and complete range of movement. When you bring the bar back, touch it to the bridge of your nose or to your forehead—not behind your head. Then push the bar back upward and slightly forward, keeping tension on the triceps at all times.

As I said, these lying triceps extensions can be done with dumbbells; however, I prefer a barbell, since it is easier to balance. In doing the exercise, I find that it is much easier to balance. Also, I find it very helpful to anchor the feet, particularly when I am using a heavy weight. If the feet aren't anchored—by a barbell, perhaps, or maybe your training partner—your whole upper body will be pulled forward by the weight on the barbell and you will find it very hard to keep your position and your balance on the bench.

Another exercise that will add shape and size to the triceps are incline triceps extensions with dumbbells—which are performed similar to the lying triceps extensions with the barbell. That is, by lying on an incline bench, raising the dumbbells up, out, and behind your head. Triceps extensions with the barbell, done in a standing position, are also good.

To do these, stand erect—if possible facing a mirror, so that you can see yourself throughout the movement. Place your feet about shoulder width apart so that you can maintain your balance easily; then press the barbell overhead and allow it to fall as far behind your head as possible, making sure that all the time you are controlling it. When you are letting the bar drop behind the head, keep your elbows pointed straight ahead so that when the bar is as far down as it will go, your elbows are pointed straight up toward the ceiling.

Another effective exercise is the one-arm triceps extension. This is probably easier to do than the barbell extension, since you are

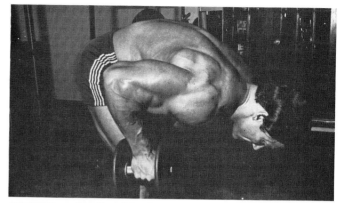

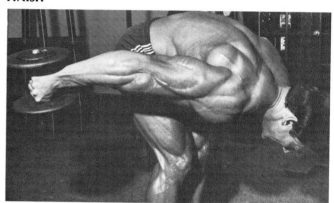

START/Dumbbell Kickback/ FINISH

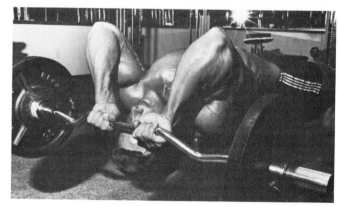

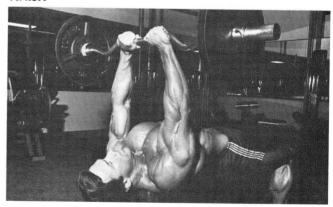

START/Lying Triceps Extension/ FINISH

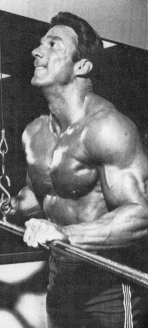

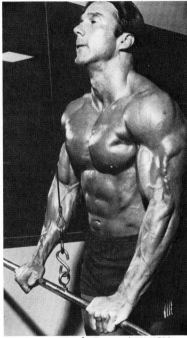

START/Lat Push-Down/ FINISH

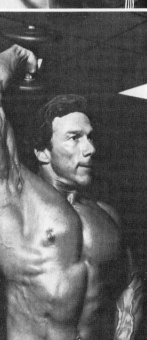

Dumbbell Triceps Extension

working one arm at a time. To do them effectively, bring the dumbbell up from your side and allow it to travel behind the head as far as possible. (You should hold the dumbbell so that the bells face straight to the front and back). By letting it go as far back as possible, you are giving the triceps a complete stretch. Throughout the movement keep your elbow straight and don't let the arm go out to the side. Then when the dumbbell is as far back as possible, your elbow will be pointed toward the ceiling.

Finally, we come to the kickback—one of my favorites. To do this, bend at the waist until the chest is resting on the upper part of the thighs. Also, try to keep your head lower than the upper part of the back. I bend slightly at the knees to take the pressure off the lower back. The kickback exercise affects the area of the lower triceps nearest the elbow, so it can be thought of as a finishing-off exercise for complete triceps work.

This is a dumbbell exercise. Holding them down toward the floor, try to get them backwards as high as you can. Each time you raise them backwards, you should lock the elbows in a stationary position and fully contract the triceps. Then bring the dumbbells slowly back to the starting position, with the bells pointed straight to the front. Be sure that every rep is done fully, locking the elbows when the dumbbells are back as far as they will go. Also, it is important that you have your arms straight throughout the exercise.

On all triceps work, I use the maximum weight I can handle. High reps and sets aren't so important; the intensity of the exercise is. As I said at the beginning, the triceps is a big muscle, capable of much hard work, so don't be afraid to really punish them. You will soon find that your arms' mass is increasing and that you are well on your way to attaining those "big arms" that, perhaps, first attracted you to bodybuilding.

Back:
How to Build It

by Robby Robinson

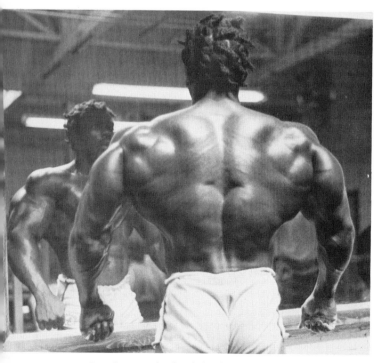

What do you think of the back development of our super-sophisticated Robby Robinson. Is there any better?

Just making muscles grow isn't what it's all about for me anymore.

When you've been blessed with the knack for gaining muscle tissue like I have, that shouldn't be a concern. What I'm saying is *I grow no matter what I do*. But size alone doesn't mean perfection in this age of super-sophisticated bodybuilders. No! Size is hardly synonymous with the aesthetic look.

The perfect *looking* physique is what we're after, so it goes without saying that huge muscles slapped carelessly onto a frame aren't a priority at my level of achievement. Indeed, size hasn't been a priority since my first Mr. Olympia disappointment in 1977. That's when size went out the window and proportion and muscular detail became vitally important to me.

I've got the size, but so what? It's the intricate details I've gradually worked into the muscle that make it freaky looking. Of all my body parts, it's the back that requires the most detail work. Man, do I love working it!

It's been said that Black bodybuilders always win Best Back, while White bodybuilders win Best Legs. To some extent, it does seem that

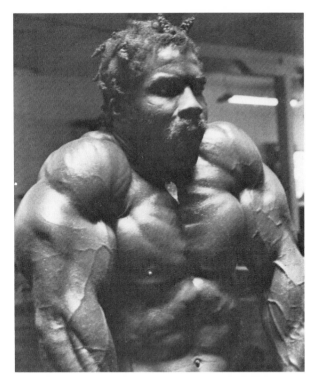

body parts are racially determined to be good or bad. For generations, Black slaves were bred to have strong backs, and I'm sure I've inherited some of this, but it still takes tremendously hard work to build a fine back. And hard work can give a scarecrow thick back muscularity. There should be no excuses for having an undeveloped back.

If you'd seen my back at the 1974 Mr. USA—my first national contest—it would have impressed you, perhaps. But it had light years to go to reach the point I've achieved now, and there's even more work needed to achieve the outer space look I'm after now.

In the May 1979 issue of *Muscle Builder* (now *Muscle & Fitness*), Joe Weider ran a color shot of my back which showed me I was getting somewhere. At the same time, that photo indicated to me how far I still am from my dream. That photo psyched me up incredibly and I'm now training my back even harder.

Variety is the key word in my back training routines. The more exercises I do and the more different ways I do the exercises, the better my back becomes. I have 20 exercises in my back training repetoire, so no part goes unworked.

Perhaps I should clarify that last statement. No part of my lats goes unworked, since I've found I need little direct lower back or trapezius training. Simply working my thigh biceps and quadriceps seems to keep my lower back in good shape, and any deltoid training bulks my trapezius sufficiently.

The only consistent thing about my back workout is that I always do it with chest as the morning half of my Monday-Wednesday-Friday Weider Double Split. Often I'll superset chest and back, while just as often I might do chest first and then back, or back and then chest. All of this depends on what I'm in the mood for when I walk into the gym at 8:30 am.

My choice of exercises also depends on my mood, but I'm careful to always do at least one for lat width (chins or pulldowns) and one for back thickness (rowing movements). This is necessary if you want to build a complete back, and only complete backs are winning contests these days.

While it may seem haphazard to constantly switch around the exercises, workout poundages, sets and reps the way I do, you must understand that I have a roadmap—and a very good one—to follow. That roadmap is the Weider Instinctive Training Principle, which I have utilized to the limit.

"Size and thickness is not enough. I had to pay attention to the smallest and most intricate details to get my back so freaky looking."
—Robby Robinson

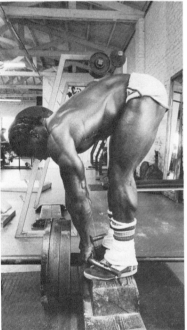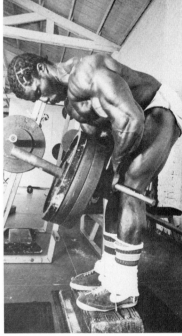

"I learned T-bar Rolls from Franco Columbu, and they're almost always in my back routine."

At this point in my bodybuilder career, I am totally in touch with my body. All I need to do is program my mind to work toward a goal, and it automatically begins making choices for me. These choices are based upon how my body feels at a particular time, where my conscious mind is, what I did the last workout, which areas are lagging or getting ahead of the others, what I've eaten, how well I've slept and scores of other bits of biofeedback.

Allowing my subconscious mind to work as a functionary of the Weider Instinctive Training Principle has been the key to my success. Instinctively, my workouts are planned to dovetail precisely with my needs at the moment, as well as with my long-range goals.

Now that all of the background is out of the way, let's go step by step through the back workout that I did this morning. It was a mind blower, and I can still feel the pump from origin to insertion in every back muscle. You wouldn't believe how good it feels, and I know that tomorrow I'll be one step closer to my goal of an outer space back.

As soon as I finished my calf work this morning, I went to the middle of the gym floor and quickly set up to do barbell bent rows. As you can see from the photos accompanying this article, I always stand on a high block as I do the rows. This allows me to stretch down fully at the bottom of the row, which gives me a greater range of motion and consequently fuller lat development.

You might also notice from the photos that I like to use a thumbless grip, which I feel is better for me. I've tried both this and a regular thumbs-around grip and have found that I get a smoother pull and better contraction at the top if my thumbs are behind the bar.

With a light poundage, I do my first set for about 20 reps, just to loosen up my back and be sure I'm warm. Then I do five sets of 12–15 reps, working the poundage up gradually in 20–30 pound jumps until I am at my peak workout weight for the final set. I am very careful, however, to keep the movement as strict as possible and to almost always use a full movement. On occasion, I will do partial reps for a different feel, since every variation counts.

My second exercise is narrow grip chins, and I am very careful to lean back on them as far as possible, since I did them more upright last week. With either style, it's very important to stretch all the way down at the bottom and then pull completely up. On the chins I did five sets

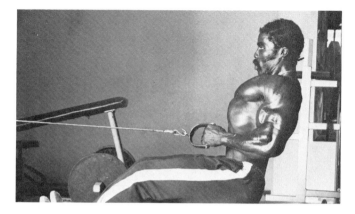

"Pulley Rows are one of the two best excercises for upper back thickness."

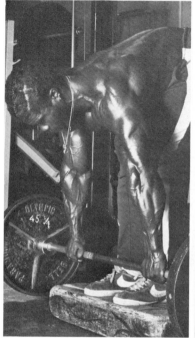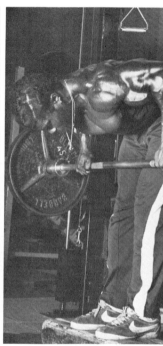

"Bent Rows are a basic thickness movement. Note how standing on a block gives me a greater stretch."

of 10–15, and then some partial reps from the top to about halfway down.

From chins, I dashed over to the seated pulley row apparatus. For my money, this is the best overall upper back movement, although I also do a lot of T-bar rows as well. On the pulley rows, I am sure to lean well into the movement when my arms are straight in order to get the maximum stretch. Then when I pull the handle in to my lower rib cage, I consciously arch my back, which allows me to fully contract the lats. Forgetting to arch is a common mistake, and I'm sure you'll quickly notice the difference once you begin arching.

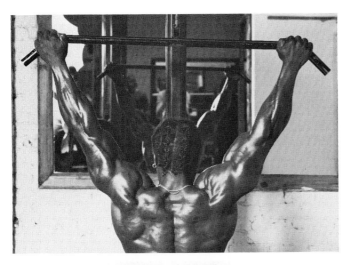

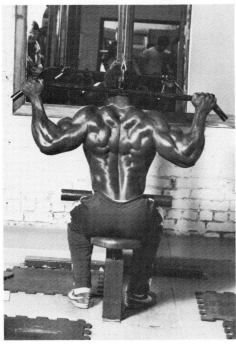

After five sets of about 12–15 reps on the pulley row, I moved on to the lat machine pulldown, more because the machine was close to the pully row than because I actually felt I needed more lat width. As I recall, I felt my pace dragging a little at that point, so I didn't want any wasted motion moving to my finishing-off exercise. I did four or five sets of 10–12 with a substantial poundage, so the restraining bar across my upper thighs was very helpful.

Since I alternate exercises as fast as possible with my training partner, these 20 sets I did for my back took only about 25 minutes, and you can believe that I was breathing like a locomotive at the conclusion of that particular workout. At the same time, though, my back was pumped to the limit. As per Joe Weider's instructions, I finished off my back with a few minutes of posing and isolation to further bring out the cuts and minute striations that are sometimes lost when you can't pose well.

I'm confident that you will profit from training your back the way I do. It's hard work, but with the variety that's built into my routine, I'm always interested in what I'm doing. That—combined with the results I'm getting—is driving me to train like a dog. It'll do the same for you!

"Lat Pulldowns and Chins are the two best excercises for back width. Be sure to pull your arms down and back."

Franco:
Updating Deltoid Training

by Dr. Franco Columbu

I haven't done a shoulder training article for many years. But with my accumulation of experience over these last few years, I think the time has come to bring you up to date on my discoveries. I will, in fact, talk about my present shoulder-training routine.

I have an entirely different approach to deltoid training today. As time went on and I became an expert on bodybuilding, I learned two important concepts that continue to elude people: 1) The importance of shoulder development to the bodybuilder; and 2) The need to understand the anatomy of the shoulder area.

Bodybuilders train their shoulders to make them big. Some succeed, and some don't. I think what set my shoulders apart from those of other bodybuilders was my relatively uncommon rear shoulder development. This development was extremely important to the posing routines that helped me win so many bodybuilding titles.

I have always worked to make my shoulders big, of course, but what's even more important perhaps, I have tried to train a "corrective" way. I trained to make the shoulders capable of supporting heavy weights.

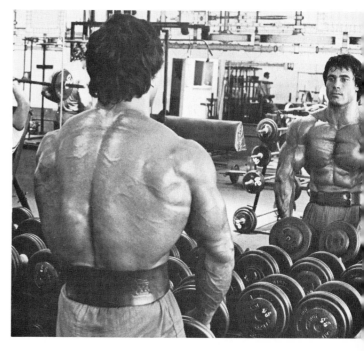

"For putting that half-cantaloupe cap on the side of the deltoids, nothing beats Side Laterals."

The shoulder is the only joint in the body supported entirely by muscles. The hip, for example, is a ball-and-socket joint, and is not wholly dependent on muscle to hold it in place.

Many bodybuilders have shoulder problems. I have observed that those who come to my office for treatment often have overdeveloped front deltoids and underdeveloped rear deltoids. This can cause the shoulder joint to go out of place anteriorly. It results from muscular imbalance, and not necessarily from weak muscles or doing an exercise that popped it out. Proper support of the shoulders means having proportionate development in the entire area.

Every upper body exercise involves the shoulder. That means you have to treat the shoulder like an axle on a car. You can have a bad tire, or even a bad steering wheel, and still be able to drive, but you cannot drive if the axle is broken. If you have a shoulder problem, it becomes almost impossible to effectively train the upper body.

I have put together a routine geared to train every part of the shoulder to a maximum degree, with maximum growth for the least amount of training time weekly.

First of all, I avoid overtraining. That took careful consideration, because I had to use heavy weights for maximum growth, strive for the maximum number of sets that would be of benefit, and gauge the capacity of each section of the shoulder. I had to be accurate to avoid overtraining. If I happened to overtrain my shoulders, the stress on them would be terrific on subsequent days when I would do heavy chest or back work.

True, I do juggle the routine, changing the number of sets and reps for different areas and different exercises, but when you grasp the concept, it all becomes simple. My purpose is to train muscles that are proportionately weaker than others. You also have to take into account that in chest and back training, some parts of the deltoid do less work than others. This means you have to compensate, working every area of the shoulder to its full potential. The development then becomes balanced.

I like to train the middle deltoid area first. I use the simple, standard exercise, Standing Lateral Raises. The torso is tilted slightly forward. As the arms are elevated to a position slightly above shoulder level, the thumbs should be pointing downward. The movement strikes the middle deltoid.

When people do these with the thumbs

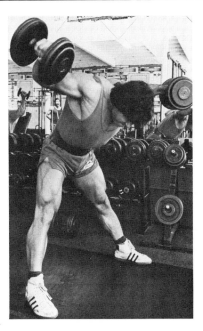

"I do a lot of Bent Laterals to balance out the rear delt."

pointing up, they are working the upper chest instead. Also, the hand should not rise above the level of the elbow. I do four sets of 10 repetitions. The first set is light, and the next three are very heavy.

Don't do them in a sitting position because the movement in that position is restricted, and you can't use weights that are heavy enough. Lateral exercises do not have to be strict; you can train heavier if you cheat a little.

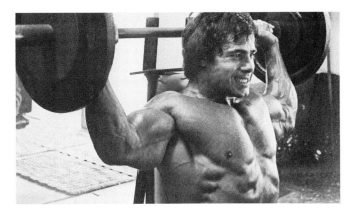

"Presses Behind The Neck are great for the whole deltoid, but you should omit them if you have a shoulder injury."

I work the rear deltoid next. The rear deltoid is usually less developed than the front. When I look at photos of other bodybuilders, the first thing I see is the lack of rear deltoid

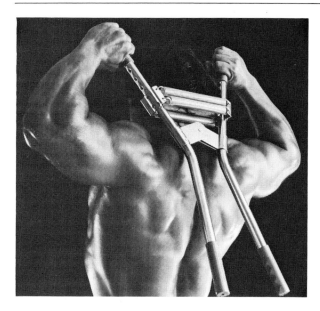

"The Super Stretch Builder is great for variety and added fun in a shoulder workout."

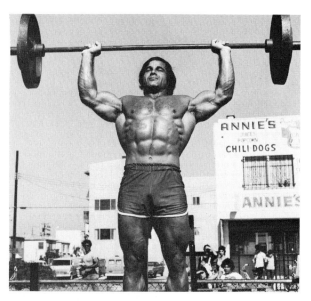

"Military Presses are the best basic delt excercise. Presses really blast the frontal deltoids."

the entire deltoid with emphasis on the front area, plus the trapezius and upper back area. One point of advice here, don't let the bar slam against the lower cervical vertebra. You might compress the nerves coming out of the spine in that area, and your shoulders will become weakened.

For your fourth exercise, do Alternate Front Dumbbell Raises, three sets of eight reps each. Raise the arm to shoulder level.

Cable Lateral Raises will be your final exercise. Here we have come full circle, returning to the middle deltoid which we worked in the first exercise. The cable movement builds width. First do one arm, then the other, raising slightly above shoulder level—three sets of 10 reps with each arm.

The foregoing program should be followed for two months. After that period, replace the cable exercise with the Standing Press, three sets of 10 reps each. Do the presses from the front.

With the Standing Press being the only change in your program, continue for the next two months. After that period, you may return to the Cable Lateral Raises again as the final exercise, dropping the press from the program.

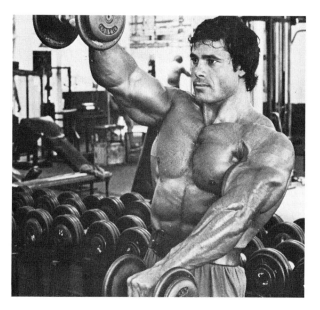

"Alternate Front Raises put the finishing touches on the anterior heads of my deltoids."

The periodic Standing Press develops the shoulder power that the other exercises won't give you. It also increases both lateral and front deltoid development. The press also enables you to work harder in the cable exercise when you return to it.

development. I look for this weakness in others because the rear deltoid happens to be one of my very strong points of development.

When the rear delt is underdeveloped, it has less supportive capability. We get back to corrective treatment here. To make up for this rear delt deficiency, do six sets of Bent-Over Lateral Raises, 10 reps each, raising the dumbbells as high as possible.

The Press Behind Neck, four sets of eight reps only, is the third exercise. This movement works

My shoulders are more developed now than ever before, mainly due to the training program I have described here. I have also recently revised my training booklets with three different programs a person can follow for the different body parts. Each program is followed for two months, and after six months you return to the first one.

This shoulder routine can be incorporated into two different training programs: (1) You can train shoulders, chest, arms and stomach the first day, and thighs, calves, back and stomach the next day; (2) You can train chest, back, thighs and calves the first day, and shoulders, arms, calves and stomach the next day.

This shoulder routine should take you no longer than 25 minutes. At that rate you can train four or five body parts in two hours, the optimum workout length.

There are people who claim they train four hours a day. I think one of the reasons I won Mr. Olympia in 1976 was because I trained two hours a day while everybody else was training four hours a day. First of all, you have to know when your body is overtrained. I have experimented with workouts of various lengths over the years, and I find I can work with maximum energy output for two hours, no more.

You don't only get good from training. You also get good from rest, relaxation and recuperation. Remember, more is not necessarily better. Two hours is better than four. In training, it's quality that counts.

"Cable Side Laterals can be substituted for Dumbbell Raises. You can also do cable laterals with the cable running across your body."

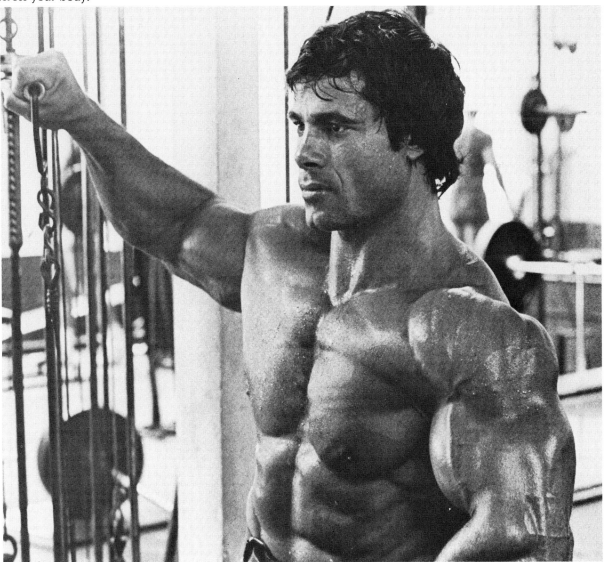

Building Muscular Thighs

by Samir Bannout
The Lion of Lebanon

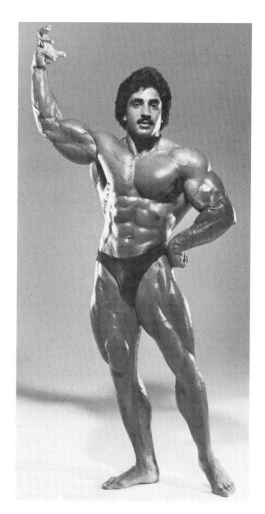

Look at those thighs!

Weak thighs and laziness go together. No wonder so many would-be champion bodybuilders languish in anonymity because of chicken-leg thighs.

The guys who are afraid of squatting are the ones who never make it. They end up looking pretty good from their belly buttons up, but from the waist down they're nowhere.

Early in my career I was the same way. At the time my upper body and calves were beginning to shape up, but my thighs were incredibly thin. My calves might actually have been bigger than my thighs at that time.

I was a good soccer and volleyball player, so the foundation for good thighs was there. Fortunately, my brother-in-law was an Olympic lifter, and he got me doing plenty of Squats.

When I started squatting, my thighs began to grow like crazy. My first basic thigh workout was 5–10 sets of full Squats, working up in weight with each set. Recently Boyer Coe told me he followed precisely the same thigh routine until well after he had won Mr. America. So you know that squatting has to be good.

Vince Gironda has condemned the Squat as an inferior thigh exercise and a superior butt builder, but I can't agree. I've squatted five reps with 500 pounds, and my butt is very small.

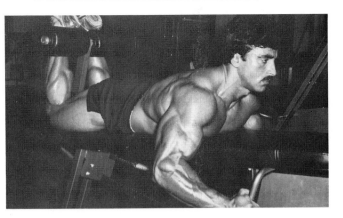

Leg Curls—Finish Position

Sergio Oliva and Arnold Schwarzenegger both squatted heavy, too, and they don't have expecially big butts.

I do my Squats with my heels elevated on a two-inch block of wood, and that puts less strain on the butt than squatting flat-footed. Still, you shouldn't be afraid of developing your buttocks, because you need some development there for the complete, masculine look.

The only thing Squats really develop is the thighs, and in my case they're doing the job almost too well. Right now my thighs are 26 1/2" in contest shape, and I could probably get them up to 28" with continued heavy squatting. But that would ruin my proportions, so I'm working more on shape and cuts.

My off-season leg workout is done twice a week, usually on Wednesdays and Saturdays. On Mondays and Thursdays I do chest and back, while Tuesdays and Fridays are reserved for shoulder and arm training. Like most competitive bodybuilders, I take Sunday off.

I always start my leg workout with about five minutes of free-hand squatting and jogging in place. I used to jump right into heavy Squats, but my right knee began to hurt. After a week's layoff, however, the problem went away and it's never come back. Now after a good warm-up, I can squat pain-free with even the heaviest weights.

Once the blood is flowing in my knees, I start my thigh workout by squatting with 135 for 25–30 reps, going up and down very quickly. Focusing my concentration on my thighs, I use a totally upright stance and place my feet no wider than shoulder width. In successive sets, I'll do 225 X 15, 315 X 12, 405 X 10 and 455 X 8.

Next I do Leg Extensions, hitting 50 X 15, 75 X 15, 95 X 15, 110 X 15 and 125 X 15. I try to do this movement very strictly and slowly, pausing at the

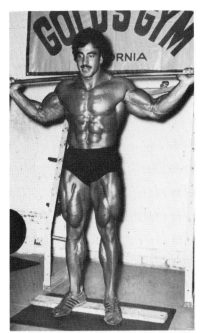

START/"Nobdy will ever build great thighs unless he's willing to do heavy Squats."/MIDPOINT

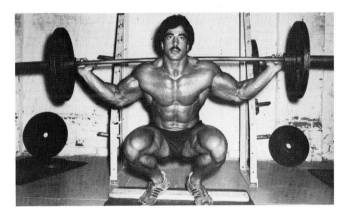

top of each rep for a full count (the Weider Peak Contraction Principle). This allows me to receive full benefit from the exercise.

As my final frontal thigh exercise, I do four sets of 10–15 reps on the Hack Slide Machine. The geometry of these machines varies quite a bit, so the weights I use would probably be meaningless to you. Suffice it to say that they are as heavy as I can go within the limits of strict form. I go for a deep burn and do all of my reps in non-lock style to take advantage of the Weider Continuous Tension Principle.

Next I move to leg biceps work, and I hit it hard, since my hamstring development has lagged at times. I'll typically do five sets: 60 X 15, 90 X 12, 110 X 10, 120 X 8 and 80 X 10–15. I use slow, continuous tension and a full range of motion. I fight to keep my hips down, and on some reps I'll even raise my shoulders at the end of a rep to accentuate the peak contraction.

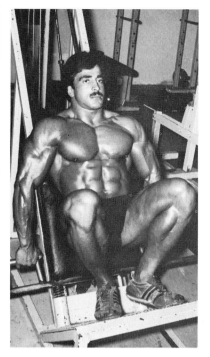
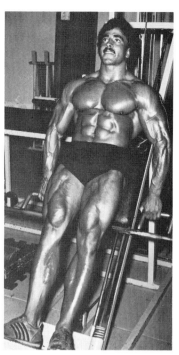

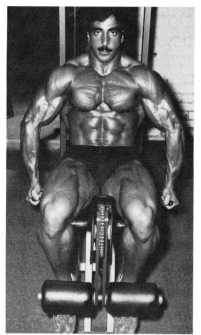
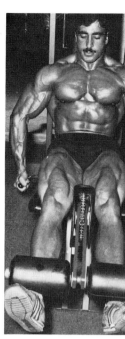

START/"I like Hack Squats for my frontal thighs, particularly the muscles just above my knees."/FINISH

START/"Leg Extentions are the most direct frontal thigh excercise in existence."/FINISH

My final thigh exercise consists of two sets of Leg Curls, using a towel and a training partner to supply the resistance. This hurts like hell because I like to work extremely hard on the negative half of the movement. Sets of 10–12 reps make my leg biceps scream for mercy.

I'll usually finish everything off with a few minutes of stretching. Sometimes this takes the form of a set of Stiff-Leg Deadlifts, but usually I do the hurdler's stretch.

All in all, it takes me about 45 minutes to train the thighs during the off-season, since I rest 45–60 seconds between sets. Including calves, abdominals and lower back, my leg-day workout lasts about 1 1/2 hours.

Pre-contest, I do basically the same workout, but I superset everything and train lighter. I also train the thighs three times a week on a double-split routine. Before a competition, I spend a lot of time tensing my thighs, and I do some wind sprints 4–5 days a week. This combination really brings out my deepest thigh cuts.

I'm often asked if it's necessary to squat heavy to develop good thighs. I don't think it's necessary—or even beneficial—to go extremely heavy like a powerlifter. You do need to squat heavy enough to limit yourself to 5–6 reps on your heaviest set, however. That's the only way you'll ever build appreciable thigh mass.

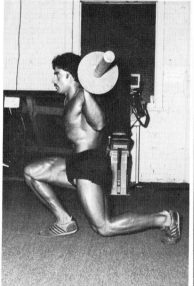
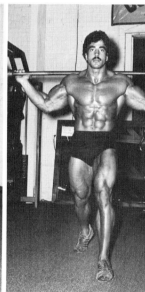

START/"Lunges are great just before a contest for cutting up the thighs."/MIDPOINT

When I was growing up in the sport, I idolized Ken Waller for his leg development, and I followed his routines published in *Muscle Builder* (now *Muscle & Fitness*). He still has the best balance between thighs and calves I've ever seen, and his hamstrings are incredible! I'd sure like to go up against him in the Olympia. If I do, I'll hit a log of leg shots.

Calves—You Can!

by Chris Dickerson

Anyone can develop a good pair of calves, and a large percentage of bodybuilders could build outstanding calves. But, unfortunately, most bodybuilders fall far short of the level of development they could attain.

I grant you that the calves are often difficult to develop. It can be boring to train them. The arms and chest are more impressive to the average person. The calves are made up of dense muscle tissue that does require high-intensity training if it's to increase in size.

However, the real problem in calf development often lies in attitude. Some bodybuilders dwell only on the negative. They think, "I can't get my calves up to the standard of Dickerson's, so why bother?"

If this is your attitude, you're beaten before you start. Even though you could build an excellent pair of calves—large, ripped, vascular, well-shaped—you don't even try. In essence, your own mental weakness denies you the chance of success!

Calf development begins with a positive mental attitude. The calves are a key muscle group, just like the shoulders. As a judge's eyes

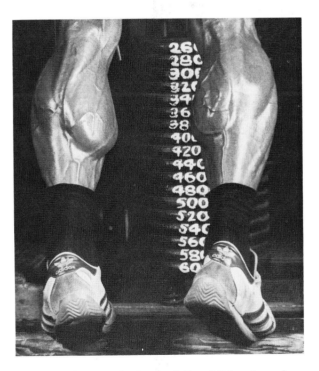

Some say the Canada Cup and Grand Prix winner has the greatest calves in bodybuilding history. Here's how he did it!

93

travel down your body, he sees the deltoids first and calves last. His opinion of your development is slanted by what he sees first and last. It's the primacy-recency concept talked about by media experts like Marshall McLuhan.

I've always placed great emphasis on leg development because, let's face it, the legs constitute half of your physique. While virtually all top bodybuilders have outstanding arm development, few have really great legs. And the ones with particularly good leg development seem to win a majority of the titles.

Heredity plays a role in how every body part eventually looks, but heredity is over-emphasized today. I've been lucky in my heredity. My calves have always been far larger than average, but at the same time I've worked extremely hard to get them up. And even though I'm quite satisfied with the way they now look, I still train them fairly hard.

I can pump my calves to over 19 inches, but when I first walked into Bill Pearl's Gym, they were three inches smaller. Even at 16 inches, however, my calves impressed the men who were training at Pearl's.

My main sports interest as a youth was soccer, and I had also taken a lot of ballet. These two activities had expanded my calves to a relatively high level before I ever touched a barbell or dumbbell. The stretching and exaggerated toe-pointing in my ballet classes was particularly beneficial.

When I decided to begin weight training I didn't know what to wear, so I showed up at Pearl's in shorts and a T-shirt. Compared to my skinny upper body, my calves must have appeared *huge!* People in the gym came running over to look at them. This confused, flustered and embarrassed me.

From the very first workout, Pearl had me on a balanced program. I devoted an equal amount of time and energy to each body part, but because of my hereditary predisposition toward lower leg development, my calves grew very quickly—too quickly!

A common error bodybuilders make is they work harder than they need to on strong points and easier than they should on weaker body parts. I fell into that trap, even though I was doing a balanced program for my entire body.

Before too long, Bill Pearl noticed what was happening and suggested I reduce my calf training. If I hadn't had Bill to coach me, I might have 20-inch calves and 16-inch arms today, and that would put my body impossibly out of

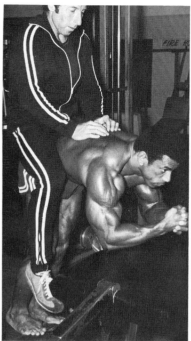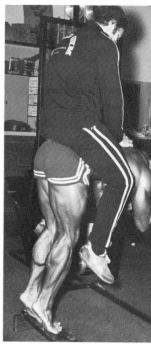

"Ed Giuliani gives me resistance for my Donkey Calf Raises. It's essential that your partner sits back as far as possible on your hips."

balance. Even the most advanced bodybuilders need coaching, so I consult with Bill Pearl frequently.

Young bodybuilders always want to know what I do for my calves. In essence, my calf training philosophy is as follows:

1. Use a variety of exercises.
2. Do very strict, full movements, exaggerating the stretch at the bottom.
3. Use high reps (25–30) and moderate weights, not low reps and heavy poundages.
4. Vary toe positions (in, straight ahead, out).
5. Do 3–5 sets per exercise and 10–15 sets per workout.
6. Train calves 4–5 times per week.
7. Train your calves first in your workout so you take advantage of the Weider Muscle Priority Training Principle.
8. Go for a deep burn on every set.

In the past I've trained my calves religiously according to the above principles. At the present time, however, I work them only twice per week with this type of program:

1. Seated Leg Press Calf
   Extension: 3–5 X 25–30 (toes out)
2. Seated Calf Machine: 3–5 X 25–30 (toes in)

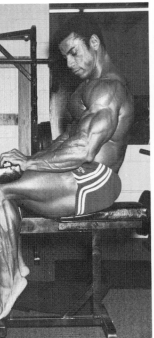 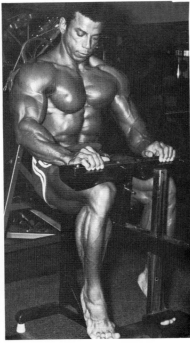

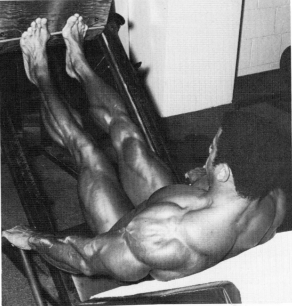

"The Seated Calf Machine movement adds width to my calves by fully developing the soleus muscle. Note how high I go up on my toes."

"Toe Presses on a Leg-Press Machine are excellent for calf definition. Only my toes and the balls of my feet are on the board."

3. Standing Calf Machine: 3–5 X 25–30
   (toes straight ahead)

I occasionally substitute Donkey Calf Raises and One-Leg Calf Raises with a dumbbell for variety. Sometimes I'll also do Calf Presses on the vertical Leg-Press Machine, but usually I prefer to do my Calf Presses seated. Regardless of the exercises used, I like to include some seated and some standing movements.

The primary reason I prefer lighter weights and higher reps is that this combination permits a longer range of motion on each movement than super-heavy weights and low reps. Too many bodybuilders get caught up in doing short and/or bouncing movements, which do little for the calves.

To get the best results, you should rise up and down on your toes fully, slowly and with maximum concentration. This will give you a deep burn very quickly, and that burn spells results.

Please note that the routine I've just given you—as well as the training philosophy I've developed—apply only to advanced bodybuilders. Beginners and intermediates should progress slowly and sensibly up to the advanced routine.

Beginners should do 3–4 sets for their calves

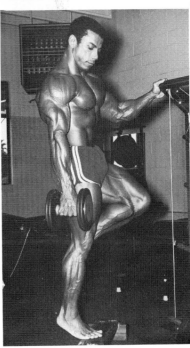

"For variety, I'll occasionally include some One-Leg Toe Raises in my program."

three times per week. Intermediates can progress up to 6–9 sets, done three or four times per week. Here is a good beginning routine:

1. Seated Calf Machine: 2 X 25–30
2. Standing Calf Machine: 2 X 25–30.

And here is an intermediate calf program that one can try:

1. Donkey Calf Raise: 3 X 25–30
2. Seated Calf Machine: 3 X 25–30
3. One-Leg Calf Raise: 3 X 25–30

Be sure to stretch fully and go for a burn on every set. Vary your toe positions and don't get carried away with using heavy weights. Sloppy reps with heavy weights won't get you far.

Work hard, be patient and you'll eventually have a very fine pair of calves to go with your overall body development. The complete body wins it, and there's absolutely no reason why you should spoil an otherwise proportionate body. If you train the calves consistently and correctly, they're bound to improve!

"On the Standing Calf Machine, I keep my legs slightly bent. But I don't allow myself to 'kick' the weight up at the finish by straightening the legs.

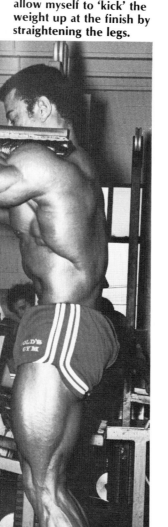

You've got to get a deep burn in the calves, which requires strict movements."

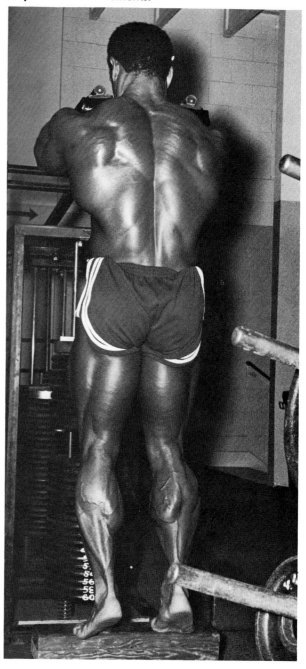

Indirect Muscle Stimulation . . . Not Training the Forearms:

Sometimes It's Better

by Mike Mentzer

Everyone has a body part—or bodyparts—that seems to grow from little or no work at all. With me, it is calves and forearms. As a matter of fact, I have noticed a certain trend to the way my body develops. It seems that the distal aspects of my musculature grow the easiest; i.e., those areas like calves and forearms, which are located the furthest distance from the center of my body. Then as you proceed towards the torso, or center, the growth of those body parts slows down. The torso itself is the slowest to respond to exercise. At times it seems that my calves and forearms grow better with little or no direct work.

Direct exercise for the forearms would be wrist curls, reverse wrist curls, reverse regular curls or Zottman curls. I have done literally no direct forearm exercise for about three years now, and yet my forearms are highly developed, perhaps my best body part. Not that my forearms don't receive a lot of work because they do, but it is never direct—always indirect.

Every time I pick up a barbell, grasp a pulley handle or latch onto a chin-up bar, I am contracting most of the muscles of the forearm. In any exercise where you must hold or grasp a piece of equipment, you will notice that the forearms become extremely fatigued and pumped, if you work the exercise intensely to a point of failure.

"I like the Wrist Curl because it stresses and stimulates the flexors and the underside of my forearm. But remember, don't overtrain the forearms—they receive benefit from indirect exercises too."

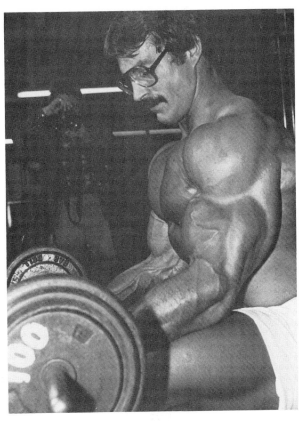

In the past two months, I have held two "special instruction week-long clinics" at George Snyder's famous Olympus Spa located in Warrington, Pa. When I tell the bodybuilders I am instructing that week, "there will be no forearm exercises included," they scoff, until I push them hard through a superset of back work, where they must grip a lat bar for two successive sets with as heavy a weight as they can handle to a point of complete muscular failure.

By the time they reach the conclusion of the second exercise of the superset, their forearms are so pumped, they have extreme difficulty holding onto the bar long enough to finish the set. That one superset is enough to convince them that any direct forearm work would be superfluous and would probably result in overtraining.

Now this is not to suggest that direct forearm exercises don't have a place in your training program. But when you take into account all of the effects they receive from other exercises, you certainly won't require much in the way of direct forearm work.

If you decide to add forearm work to your routine, limit it to a few exercises for only a couple of intense sets carried to failure. Two exercises that I like—together they more or less work the entire forearm—are wrist curls and reverse curls. The wrist curls will stress and stimulate the flexors and the underside of your forearm, while the reverse curls work primarily the extensors and the meaty radialis muscles along with the flexors. I would suggest you limit yourself to two weekly forearm workouts on your upper arm days following biceps work.

A SUMMARY OF FOREARM TRAINING TIPS

1. Do not overtrain your forearms. They receive a lot of benefit from many of the "indirect exercises" you do.
2. Use heavy weights that allow up to ten reps and train them to failure; do not stop any set at an arbitrary number of reps. Go to failure!
3. Train your forearms only once or twice a week.
4. Train them on the day you work upper arms following the upper arm workout. This should be at the end of your training session, otherwise your fatigued forearms will become a weak link in training your torso.
5. Include exercises that work the entire forearm, the flexors on the bottom of the forearm and the extensors located on the top of the forearm.

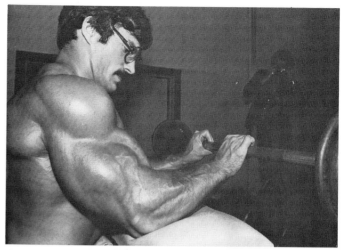
"The reverse Wrist Curl does wonders for the extensors and the meaty radialis muscles along with the flexors. Keep the forearms stationary in this movement."

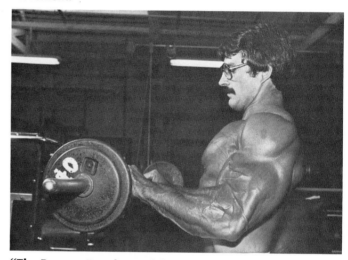
"The Reverse Regular Curl, besides working the forearms, gives the brachialis on the outside of the upper arm good stimulation."

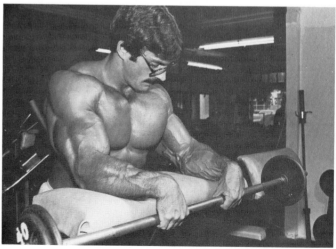
"Just the constant gripping of the bar in a grueling workout is enough to pump the forearms to the extreme."

The Ripped Waistline

by Danny Padilla

When I first started bodybuilding, everyone who was supposed to know anything about the sport told me that no one who was very tall or very short (guess which category I fall into!) could develop great abdominals. And for much of my bodybuilding career, like a jerk I believed them.

My abs were far below average until after I'd won both Mr. America and Mr. Universe, and embarked on my professional bodybuilding career. At that point it became obvious that I'd have to sharpen them up if I was ever going to stand a chance of winning Mr. Olympia.

Three years ago I embarked on an abdominal reclamation program that brought them up so rapidly that within a year my abs were one of my best body parts. Now all I need to do is stay on a maintenance schedule most of the year and then kick in a version of my ab specialization workout for six weeks while peaking for a contest.

In this article I'll outline this specialization routine, plus give you my maintenance program. I think you'll get the same type of results I got. Or perhaps you'll do even better, because I'm not particularly blessed with the genetic potential for great abdominal development.

There are several rules you must follow to get good abdominal thickness and muscularity. They are:

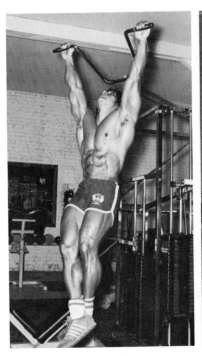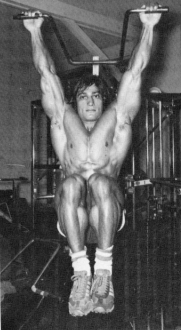

LEG RAISES/"Hanging Leg Raises and Knee Raises blitz and rip my lower abdominals."

99

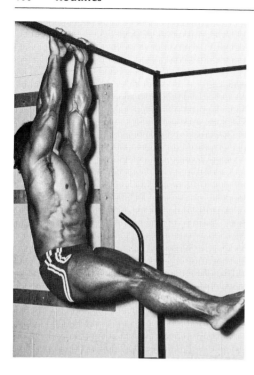

1. Train the abdominals 5–7 times per week, even during the off-season. Before a contest, you can even train them twice a day.

2. For maximum abdominal definition, you'll definitely have to diet for several weeks prior to a competition.

3. Do the greatest variety of exercises possible. This makes the workouts less boring and gives you better all-round midsection development.

4. Keep the reps high (at least 25 on each movement, and as many as 100 per exercise).

5. Do the reps with a fairly fast cadence, and be sure to use a full range of motion on each exercise.

6. Rest as little as possible between movements. An abdominal routine should be one big Giant Set (take it from The Giant Killer).

7. Schedule your abs first in your workout because ab training is an excellent warm-up for the rest of the body. Also, if your abs are weak, you should be doing them first, a la the Weider Muscle Priority Principle.

8. Be persistent and work out regularly.

Okay, now we can move on to my specialization routine for abdominals. There are two parts to it. I did the two parts on alternate days, Monday through Saturday. If on occasion I felt particularly energetic on Sundays, I'd hit another ab workout on that day (normally I take a complete day off from training on Sunday).

Below is the routine. Do each part with no rest between exercises.

Part A
1. Roman Chair Sit-Ups: 4 X 25–50
2. Seated Twisting: 4 X 50–100
3. Hanging Knee Raises: 4 X 25–30
4. Side Bends (no weight): 4 X 50–100
5. Crunches: 4 X 25

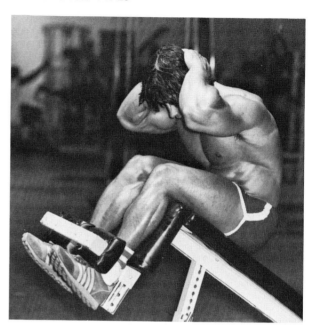

INCLINE SIT-UPS/"This was the only upper-ab movement I did until three years ago."

Part B
1. Incline Sit-Ups: 4 X 25
2. Seated Twisting: 4 X 50–100
3. Hanging Leg Raises: 4 X 15–20
4. Side Bends (no weight): 4 X 50–100
5. Rope Pulldowns (on lat machine): 4 X 25–30

In my maintenance program, I do about half as many sets, but I still train my abdominals six times per week at the start of each workout. Here's a typical maintenance routine:

Part A
1. Roman Chair Sit-Ups: 3 X 25–50
2. Side Bends (no weight): 3 X 50–100
3. Crunches: 3 X 25–30
4. Seated Twisting: 3 X 50–100

Part B
1. Hanging Knee Raises: 3 X 25–30
2. Side Bends (no weight): 3 X 50–100
3. Rope Pulldowns: 3 X 25–30
4. Seated Twisting: 3 X 50–100

The specialization workout took about 30–35

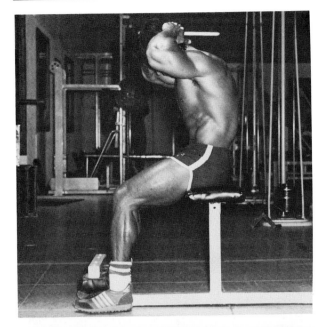

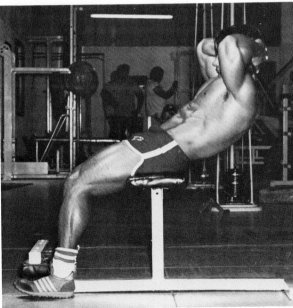

ROMAN CHAIR SIT-UPS/"Then I discovered Roman Chair Sit-Ups, which are super for the top two rows of abdominal muscles."

minutes each day. That's a lot, but the results were so good I didn't mind the boredom. The maintenance workout should take no more than 20 minutes.

Both of these workouts are pretty stiff for a beginning or intermediate bodybuilder, so let me offer the following alternative routines for less experienced athletes.

Beginners (three times per week)
1. Sit-Ups: 3 X 25–50
2. Leg Raises: 3 X 25–50
3. Seated Twisting: 3X 50–100

Intermediates (4–5 times per week)
1. Sit-Ups: 3 X 25–50
2. Hanging Knee Raises: 3 X 25–30
3. Crunches: 3 X 25–30
4. Side Bend or Twisting: 3 X 50–100

Stay on these simple routines, and you'll soon progress to the advanced level and eventually to competition. I think as you increase the intensity of your training, you'll likely find that your abs progress much faster than the rest of your body. If you have the potential, you can develop a washboard ab structure in only 6–8 months.

If you're simply an average person seeking to reduce your waistline, you'll find these exercises will work effectively for you as well. Be careful, however, to maintain a reduced-calorie diet, because you'll never make much progress in tightening your waist if you persist in stuffing it.

I know all this sounds pretty simple, but sometimes the simplest routines are the most effective. So think positively and go for it!

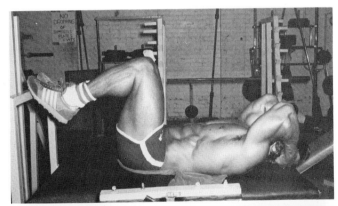

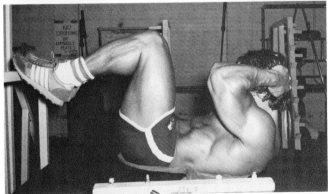

CRUNCHES/"This short movement works the entire frontal abdomen, but particularly the upper abs."

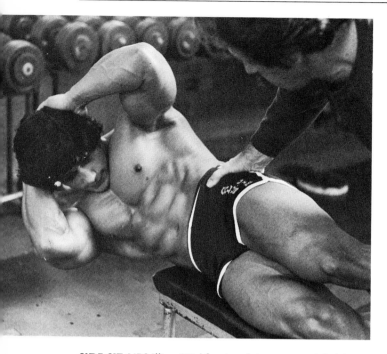

SIDE SIT-UPS/"Joe Weider taught me a special Side Sit-Up that ripped and striated my intercostals and obliques like no other exercise I've ever done."

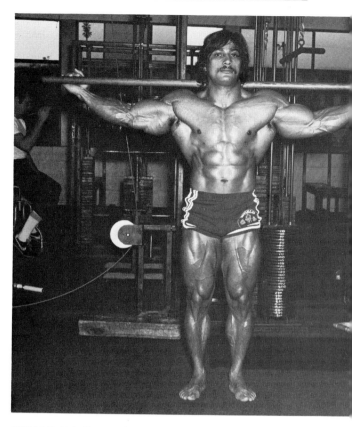

SIDE BENDS/"From this position I bend rhythmically to each side as far as I can to shape my external obliques."

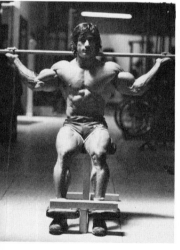
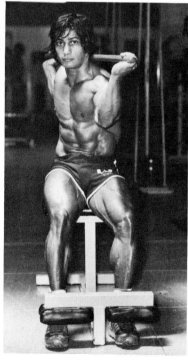

SEATED TWISTING/"I like doing Twists seated instead of standing because the seated position keeps my hips motionless."

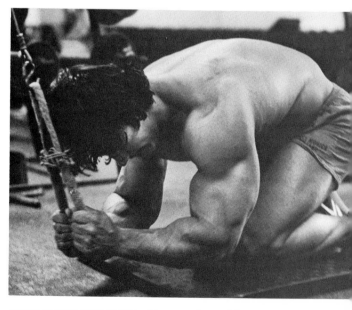

ROPE PULLDOWNS/"Nothing can beat this movement for developing a great serratus-intercostal tie-in."

Power Exercises for Bodybuilders

by Joe Weider

Many of the world's most massive bodybuilders did power exercises. Arnold Schwarzenegger was a former European champion weightlifter. Sergio Oliva was a weightlifting champ in Cuba. Franco Columbu is a living, breathing hydraulic hoist.

Frank Zane saw the light and incorporated powerlifting in his training for the 1979 Mr. Olympia. It gave him the mass he needed to win the title for the third time. The Mentzer brothers and Casey Viator do Power Cleans and Deadlifts as part of their bodybuilding routine. The heavy lifting he did over a three-year period played a big part in Chris Dickerson's sensational comeback in 1979.

Most bodybuilders today, however, are depending too much on machines, benches and other contrivances. Some of the equipment serves the bodybuilding purpose. Yet, the gimmick trend seems to be creating a generation of bodybuilders with impressive muscles but insufficient strength.

Power movements are the most important and basic part of training routine. The bodybuilders of the '40s and '50s were still doing those movements, vestiges of the early weightlifting ethic in training. They were rugged—and looked it—those first bodybuilding champs like Clancy Ross, Armand Tanny and Roy Hilligenn.

As time went by, however, power movements fell out of fashion because they didn't accentuate development of isolated muscle groups, not in the way that Incline Curls or Concentration Curls could build big, showy biceps, for example.

The competitive bodybuilders must be blamed for this lapse because they are the ones who set the style. They concentrate on building individual muscle groups, and the end product looks like it has been put together by a stone mason rather than a sculptor. By that I mean that the norm today is the massive, peaked biceps, a skinny waistline and weak haunches. In short, most of today's bodybuilders are not proportionately developed.

It goes without saying that individual body parts must be worked separately, using any equipment that effectively builds them. But for muscle to give the ultimate effect, it must be built on a solid foundation.

One might call this the "layered effect" in bodybuilding. Muscle must have a strong base to support its superstructure. In order to build the ultimate body, the overall power must be established. Overall power enables the bodybuilder to handle heavier weights in all specialization exercises. It lays the foundation for building lasting muscular size and strength. But absolute power can be developed only through power exercises.

One of the few power exercises that has survived to the present is the Squat. The basic leg movement, the Squat builds size and power. But at best it remains a token exercise for the majority of bodybuilders. They excuse themselves from extensive squatting on the grounds that it might thicken their waist, broaden their hips or make their thighs "too big."

So they turn to the machines, replacing Squats with Leg Extensions or Horizontal Leg Presses, trusting these movements will give them the desired development. When the development lags, they'll do more of the same exercises, subjecting their knees to excessive stress because of the rigid nature of the machines.

When properly done, the free-weight Squat, with its natural checks and balances, causes no knee stress. The effort is distributed throughout the body, and it's this distribution that makes you stronger on all other exercises.

Every bodybuilder should do Squats. Later in this article I'll outline a few other movements that I hope all bodybuilders will incorporate into their routines. These movements work for other body parts in the same way that the Squat works for the legs. They build *total* body power, while laying solid muscle on specific bodyparts.

One impressive feature that characterizes the bodybuilding star is the deep tie-in between his massively developed traps and deltoids. It gives the appearance of ruggedness and power. Another feature is the deep gorge between the erector spinae muscles of the back, most evident on luminaries like Franco Columbu, Casey Viator and Roy Callender. In the cases of all three men, powerful glutes support their impressive upper body structures.

I don't think this type of development can be accomplished without using power movements. Bodybuilders today no longer clean weights from the floor to the shoulder for overhead pressing. They start their barbell exercises with takeoffs from special racks. Flat, incline and decline benches have also worked their way into the bodybuilding routine, making the torso itself a rather inert mass practically divorced from the arm and shoulder action.

To avoid this disassociation and to integrate the body, the bodybuilder should include two power exercises in each workout. With four of these exercises to choose from, he can alternate, doing two one day and the other two the next.

Warm up with a light weight before doing these exercises in earnest. If you have never done them before, they may feel awkward. So don't do them explosively with high poundages. Take a few weeks to get the feel of them, concentrating on doing them fast, smoothly and rhythmically. Each of these movements calls a great part of the total body musculature into play. Moments after you finish a set of reps, you'll get a sudden rush of heavy breathing that will last about two minutes. This rush is known as the cardiovascular effect. Power movements will give you plenty of it.

After the warm-up, handle a weight that allows you to do nine repetitions. Take a couple minutes rest, then do a second set with a heavier poundage that allows you seven reps. Rest again, then do a third set with a poundage that allows five reps. Three sets should be enough.

Handle as heavy a weight as you can without straining. In the beginning, use moderate weights. After you have become coordinated and conditioned, handle heavy weights, forcing out the last couple of reps.

Don't superset these movements. Take a good rest (about three minutes) between sets so that you can exert full power on successive sets.

1. **Power Snatches**—Grip the bar, using the snatch grip, hands more than shoulder width apart. Without bending the knees or moving the feet, power snatch the weight to arms' length overhead. Lower the weight below the knees and repeat. Don't let the weight touch the floor until you have completed the required reps.

2. **Power Cleans**—Use a shoulder-width grip. Stand close to the bar, knees bent, hips lower than the shoulders, and head up. Pull the weight up as high and fast as possible (keeping it close to the body), then whip the elbows under the bar, catching the bar at the shoulders. Lower the bar to a position below the knees and repeat, using the same starting position. Don't let the weight touch the floor until you have finished the reps.

3. **One-Arm High Pulls**—With heels about 15 inches apart, grip a dumbbell, resting on the floor between the feet. Keep the other hand away from the body. At the start of the pull with knees bent, keep the hips lower than the shoulders and the head up. Pull the dumbbell to shoulder level, coming to a fully erect position. Without pausing, lower the weight again to the starting position, without letting the weight actually touch the floor. Use a swing-time motion with no pauses at the top or bottom.

Don't let the weight touch the floor until you have completed the reps. After doing the required number with one arm, do the required number with the other arm.

4. **One-Arm Side Presses**—Bring a heavy weight to the shoulder, using both arms if necessary. After the weight is balanced at the shoulder, take away the free hand, and by leaning away from the weight, press the weight overhead. Lower the weight to the shoulder and repeat for the required number of reps. Do one arm first, then the other. The forearm should be vertical as the elbow and triceps rest against the lats at the start of the press.

Do one of the two-arm movements and one of the one-arm movements per workout. These power movements develop areas otherwise neglected by ordinary bodybuilding exercises. The interaction of many muscles at once forces heavier loads on muscles or areas that have never had to undergo such stress. Power Snatches and Cleans build the upper and lower back quickly because of the heavy poundages. One-Arm High Pulls and One-Arm Presses build the deltoid and other muscles of the shoulder girdle and back more completely. Areas bypassed by lighter bodybuilding exercises will feel the full force of these heavier movements.

There are other power exercises you can do, such as Deadlifts, Two-Arm Dumbbell Cleans, One-Arm Swings, and Two-Arm Swings. But for now, if you stick with the routine I've described here, it will get you going on the road to all-around strength and power.